Hospice/Palliative Care Training

UNIPAC Three: *Assessment and Treatment of Pain in the Terminally Ill*

Authors

Porter Storey, M.D.
Clinical Associate Professor of Medicine and Assistant Professor of Family Medicine
Baylor College of Medicine

Consultant in Neuro-Oncology and Adjunct Assistant Professor of Medicine
University of Texas MD Anderson Cancer Center

Medical Director
The Hospice at the Texas Medical Center

Carol F. Knight, Ed.M.
Hospice Education Consultant

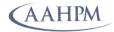

American Acadmy of Hospice an Palliative Medicine

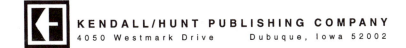

KENDALL/HUNT PUBLISHING COMPANY
4050 Westmark Drive   Dubuque, Iowa 52002

Copyright ©1997 by the American Academy of Hospice and Palliative Medicine
4700 W. Lake Avenue
Glenview, IL 60025-1485

ISBN 0-7872-1938-X

All rights reserved, including that of translation into other languages. No part of this publication may be reproduced or transmitted in any form or by any means, electronic or mechanical, including photocopying, recording, or any information storage and retrieval system, without permission in writing from the copyright holder.

Printed in U.S.A.
10 9 8 7 6 5 4 3 2

Acknowledgments

The authors and the American Academy of Hospice and Palliative Medicine are deeply grateful to the following reviewers for their participation in the development of this UNIPAC. Their extensive comments and thoughtful suggestions greatly improved its contents.

We want to express special gratitude to the reviewers for coordinating local testing of the UNIPAC and to all the practicing physicians, fellows, residents, and medical students who participated in the field-testing.

Reviewers

Julia L. Smith, M.D.
Assistant Professor of Oncology in Medicine
University of Rochester Cancer Center

Medical Director
Genesee Region Home Care/Hospice
Rochester, New York

John W. Finn, M.D.
Medical Director
Hospice of Michigan
Southfield, Michigan

Gerald H. Holman, M.D.
Chief of Staff
Veterans Administration Medical Center
Amarillo, Texas

Eli N. Perencevich, D.O.
Clinical Assistant Professor of Medicine
Ohio State University

Medical Director
Hospice of Columbus
Columbus, Ohio

The American Academy of Hospice and Palliative Medicine's Self Study Training Program

The self-study program, *Hospice/Palliative Care Training for Physicians*, is under development by the American Academy of Hospice and Palliative Medicine and is made possible with federal funds from the National Cancer Institute's Cancer Education Grant Program, Grant # CA66771-02. The Academy recognizes a need for physician training materials on hospice/palliative care and has designed the self-study program to meet its own education goals, as well as those of the National Cancer Institute. The program consists of multiple modules, or UNIPACs, each of which follows the recommended format for self-instructional learning and includes behavioral objectives, a pretest, reading material, clinical situations for demonstrating knowledge application, a posttest, and references.

UNIPACs currently being developed include (1) The Hospice/Palliative Approach to Caring for the Terminally Ill, (2) Psychological, Spiritual, and Physiological Aspects of Dying and Bereavement, (3) Assessment and Treatment of Pain in the Terminally Ill, (4) Management of Selected Nonpain Symptoms in the Terminally Ill, (5) Caring for the Terminally Ill: Communication and the Interdisciplinary Team Approach, and (6) Ethical and Legal Decision Making When Caring for the Terminally Ill.

Although the UNIPACs may be used by candidates when reviewing for the written examination of the American Board of Hospice and Palliative Medicine, they were not developed for that purpose. The Academy recommends that candidates also review basic information in the field of hospice/palliative medicine that can be found in a number of excellent resources.

The information presented and opinions expressed herein are those of the authors and do not necessarily represent the views of the sponsor or its parent agencies, the National Institutes of Health, the United States Public Health Service, the reviewers, or a consensus of the members of the American Academy of Hospice and Palliative Medicine. Any recommendations made by the authors must be weighed against the physician's own clinical judgment, based on but not limited to such factors as the patient's condition, benefits versus risks of suggested treatment, and comparison with recommendations of pharmaceutical compendia and other authorities.

The American Academy of Hospice and Palliative Medicine is accredited by the Accreditation Council for Continuing Medical Education (ACCME) to sponsor continuing medical education for physicians and therefore designates this CME activity for three (3) credit hours in Category 1 of the Physician's Recognition Award of the American Medical Association.

For information on the availability of specific UNIPACs and other Academy materials, please contact the American Academy of Hospice and Palliative Medicine at (352) 377-8900.

Assessment and Treatment of Pain in the Terminally Ill

Table of Contents

About UNIPAC Three: *Assessment and Treatment of Pain in the Terminally Ill* . . **1**
    Introduction to the UNIPAC 2
    Pretest 3
    Behavioral Objectives 5
    Introduction to Pain Management 5

Principle One: *Assess for Multiple Causes of Pain* **7**
    Introduction to Assessment 8
    Assess for Multiple Causes of Pain 8
    Assess For Pain Caused by Noncancer-related Physical Conditions 11
    Assess for Cancer-related Physical Pain 12
    Assess For Nonphysical Causes of Pain 12
    Clinical Situation Illustrating the Assessment of Multiple Causes of Pain   15

Principle Two: *Treat Each Type of Pain* **19**
    Introduction to Treatment 20
    Treat Pain Caused by Noncancer-related Physical Conditions 20
    Treat Cancer-related Physical Pain 21
    Treat Nonphysical Causes of Pain 41
    Continuing Clinical Situation Illustrating the Treatment 45
        of Multiple Causes of Pain

Principle Three: *Reassess When Pain is Uncontrolled* **51**
    Introduction to Reassessment 52
    Reassess for Total Pain 52
    Reassess Need for Increased Involvement of Interdisciplinary Team 52
    Reassess Patient Compliance 53
    Reassess Need for Increased Dosages 53
    Reassess Need for Alternative Routes of Drug Administration 54
    Reassess Need for Involvement of Other Medical Specialists 57

Review Clinical Situation **59**

Test Clinical Situation **69**
    Correct Responses 74

Pretest Correct Responses **76**

Posttest **78**

References **82**

Posttest Answer Sheet—Removable

Tables 2 and 9 Reference Cards—Removable

Tables

Tables

Table 1	Four Components of Total Pain	13
Table 2	Oral Morphine Equivalents	26
Table 3	Conversion of Oral Opioid Doses to Parenteral Doses	28
Table 4	Starting Doses for Opioid-naive Patients	30
Table 5	Initial Opioid Doses for Children	31
Table 6	Titration Increments for Opioid Dosing	32
Table 7	Drugs and Routes to Avoid in Hospice/Palliative Care	33
Table 8	An Effective Step-wise Bowel Regimen	35
Table 9	Suggested Adjuvant Drug Dosages	40

About UNIPAC Three

Assessment and Treatment of Pain in the Terminally Ill

- Introduction to the UNIPAC
  - Purpose
  - Recommended Procedure
  - Continuing Medical Education

- Pretest

- Behavioral Objectives

- Introduction to Pain Management
  - Three Basic Principles of Pain Management
    - Assess for the Multiple Causes of Pain
    - Treat Each Type of Pain
    - Reassess When Pain is Uncontrolled

About UNIPAC Three: *Assessment and Treatment of Pain in the Terminally Ill*

Introduction to the UNIPAC

Purpose

A UNIPAC is a self-instructional training program. This UNIPAC describes three basic principles of pain control and presents specific, practical information designed to help physicians assess and manage pain in terminally ill patients. Clinical situations likely to be encountered on an almost daily basis are included to illustrate the application of specific principles.

Additional information is available from the American Academy of Hospice and Palliative Medicine, whose staff can direct you to physicians specializing in palliative medicine who are more than willing to share their experiences with the management of pain.

Recommended Procedure

To receive maximum benefit from this module the following procedure is recommended:

- Complete the pretest before reading the module.
- Review the behavioral objectives.
- Study each section and the accompanying clinical situation.
- Study the review clinical situation.
- Complete the test clinical situation and compare your responses with those on the answer sheet.
- Study the correct responses to the pretest.
- Complete the posttest by marking your answers on the answer sheet.

Continuing Medical Education

The American Academy of Hospice and Palliative Medicine designates this CME activity for three (3) credit hours in Category 1 of the Physician's Recognition Award of the American Medical Association. To receive CME credit for completing this UNIPAC, please follow the instructions on the Posttest Answer Sheet at the back of this publication.

Pretest

Before proceeding, please complete the following true/false items. The correct responses are included at the end of the UNIPAC.

	T	F
1) Patients usually describe neuropathic pain as shooting, burning, or stabbing.		
2) The correct dose of oral morphine provides effective relief from pain in most terminally ill patients.		
3) Meperidine (Demerol) often is the analgesic of choice in the hospice/palliative care setting.		
4) Morphine usually relieves neuropathic pain without the use of adjuvant drugs.		
5) Clinically significant respiratory depression is a common result of opioid use.		
6) Subcutaneous infusion is an effective route for delivering morphine to patients unable to swallow.		
7) A history and physical exam are the most important first steps in the assessment process.		
8) An effective dose of immediate-release oral morphine provides about 4 hours of pain relief.		
9) All terminally ill patients with depression should receive pharmacological treatment.		
10) Most patients receiving opioid therapy should be placed on a laxative regimen.		
11) When titrating morphine, the total daily dose should be increased by only 25% each day.		
12) Small doses of antidepressants can help relieve neuropathic pain.		

About UNIPAC Three: *Assessment and Treatment of Pain in the Terminally Ill*

Pretest *(continued from page 3)*

	T	F
13) To calculate the initial dose of subcutaneous hydromorphone (Dilaudid), divide the patient's dose of oral morphine by 20.		
14) Effective pain management is dependent on an effective assessment of the causes of noncancer-related pain, cancer-related pain, and nonphysical pain.		
15) One oxycodone and acetaminophen (Percocet) tablet is roughly equivalent to 5 mg of oral morphine.		
16) Booster doses of opioids to relieve breakthrough pain should be prescribed in doses that are about 1/2 of the regular 4-hour dose.		
17) Bone pain is often described as tender, deep, and aching.		
18) Visceral spasm pain can be effectively treated with an opioid and an anticholinergic, such as scopolamine.		
19) Soluble tablets can provide effective sublingual delivery of morphine.		
20) Hospice/palliative care can relieve physical, emotional, social, *and* spiritual pain.		

Behavioral Objectives

Upon completion of this UNIPAC, a physician should be able to demonstrate the ability to:

- Assess for the presence of cancer-related and noncancer-related pain.
- Identify social, emotional, and spiritual pain.
- Differentiate bone, neuropathic, and visceral pain.
- Prescribe appropriate adjuvant drugs to treat bone, neuropathic and visceral pain, and pain due to raised intracranial pressure.
- Calculate oral morphine equivalents of codeine, oxycodone, and hydromorphone.
- Calculate a continuous subcutaneous-infusion dose of morphine and hydromorphone.
- Calculate an appropriate starting dose of morphine therapy for an opioid-naive patient.
- Prescribe an appropriate alternative route of drug administration.
- Prescribe appropriate treatments for nausea and constipation associated with opioid use.

Introduction to Pain Management

Despite the publication of hundreds of articles on the assessment and treatment of pain, many dying patients continue to suffer from unrelieved pain during their last months of life. Of cancer patients with pain, 40% to 50% report moderate to severe pain, and 25% to 30% describe their pain as very severe.[1]

Most terminally ill patients experience several different types of pain. Twycross found that 80% of advanced cancer patients suffered from more than one type of pain and 34% experienced four or more types of pain, each of which demanded a different set of treatments.[2] It has been estimated that at least 25% of all cancer patients die without adequate pain relief.[2]

Because most pain experienced during the terminal phases of life can be managed using relatively simple techniques, the question remains, why do so many patients continue to suffer?

A recent article illustrates this point. A group of AIDS patients who were hospitalized with intractable pain received daily physician visits, but their pain remained uncontrolled. A specialized pain team was asked to consult and, after assessing the patients, the team ordered oral morphine on a 24-hour around-the-clock schedule. The results of opioid therapy were described as dramatic, and most of the patients experienced relief from their pain.[3]

Prescribing oral morphine on a 24-hour around-the-clock schedule is one of the most basic techniques of pain control. Why are specialized pain teams often needed to initiate such fundamental techniques? Possible reasons include the following:

- Continued physician unfamiliarity with pain assessment and treatment
- Continued belief in misconceptions about morphine
- Undue concern about addiction issues, regulatory body reprimands, and lawsuits concerning the use of opioids

Three Basic Principles of Pain Management

Cancer pain can be managed effectively in up to 90% of patients[1] by following the basic principles of effective pain management and by using relatively simple pain management techniques.

Effective pain management is a continuous three-step process, the first step being a thorough assessment of all types of pain the patient is experiencing. The second step is treating each type of pain with individualized, type-specific interventions, and the third step involves continuous reassessment of the patient's pain and the efficacy of prescribed treatments. When pain increases or remains uncontrolled, a thorough assessment is reinstituted and type-specific treatments are prescribed until all types of pain are adequately controlled.

The three basic principles of pain management are:

ONE: Assess for multiple causes of pain

TWO: Treat each type of pain

THREE: Reassess continuously, especially when pain remains uncontrolled

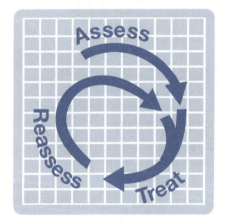

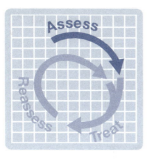

Principle One

Assess for Multiple Causes of Pain

- Introduction to Assessment
- Assess for Multiple Causes of Pain
  - Assess Pain from Three Sources
  - Use Pain Assessment Scales
  - Remember the Needs of Special Populations
  - Listen During the Assessment Process

- Assess for Pain Caused by Noncancer-related Physical Conditions

- Assess for Cancer-related Physical Pain
- Assess for Nonphysical Causes of Pain

- Clinical Situation Illustrating the Assessment of Multiple Causes of Pain

Introduction to Assessment

Many dying patients experience *total pain*—a combination of four different types of pain, each of which interacts with the others and can result in all-encompassing pain or suffering. The four components of total pain are:

- Physical pains, usually multiple
- Emotional or psychic pain
- Social or interpersonal pain
- Spiritual or existential pain

When assessing for multiples causes of pain, the first step in the assessment process is to complete a careful history and physical, maneuvers that are most likely to reveal important information about the patient's pain without causing additional pain and expense.

An effective assessment employs careful listening, open-ended questioning, and the use of individualized patient-completed pain assessment scales to correctly identify each pain's location, intensity, and etiology. This section of the UNIPAC discusses the assessment of the following sources of pain:

- Physical pain caused by noncancer-related conditions such as arthritis or decubiti
- Physical pain caused by cancer-related conditions such as nerve damage or bone involvement
- Nonphysical pain caused by conditions such as anxiety, isolation, and loss of meaning

Assess for Multiple Causes of Pain

A complete assessment is the essential first step in pain management—it is the building block upon which rests effective pain management. Assessments should include a history, physical, and the use of a numerical or visual analogue pain assessment scale—all tools that encourage patient communication about each pain's location, intensity, and etiology regardless of source. Laboratory, radiographic, and imaging studies may also be useful, but they are not a substitute for a thorough and compassionate assessment interview.

Assess Pain from Three Sources

- Assess for pain caused by non-cancer-related physical conditions.
- Assess for different types of cancer-related physical pain.
- Assess for nonphysical causes of pain.

Although a complete assessment may take an hour or two, it is time well spent. During the initial assessment process, correctly identifying the type and severity of pain from each source results in more immediate provision of appropriate treatments and more rapid relief from pain. Hurried, incomplete assessments often fail to identify the presence of multiple causes of pain, such as neuropathic pain *and* spiritual pain, in which case the patient's unidentified spiritual agony may interfere with efforts to relieve the patient's equally severe neuropathic pain. During the assessment process it is also important to determine the efficacy of current analgesic prescriptions.

Use Pain Assessment Scales

Although pain assessment scales can be time-consuming to complete and, in some cases, may be viewed by the patient as an imposition, the use of patient-completed scales is invaluable, particularly when difficulties with verbal communication affect the patient's ability to adequately report pain and when concerns arise about the efficacy of ongoing pain control measures. The results obtained on numerical scales can be used in outcome studies to determine the effectiveness of various pain control measures.[4]

The use of a specific type of scale is less important than ensuring the scale is:

- Completed by the patient rather than by an observer
- Flexible enough to be adapted to the needs of a particular patient
- Simple enough to be used regularly
- Used consistently with the patient

Adapting the scale to each patient is vital. Children may respond to a series of "smiley" faces and patients from other specific populations may find it easier to respond to individualized symbols for pain, for instance a series of pictures of fire that are larger and larger. Regardless which scale is used, it is important to continue using the same scale with the same patient to ensure reliability.

Remember the Needs of Special Populations

Children, patients from other cultures, and patients with HIV disease are three population groups that require extra care during the assessment process.

Children and Patients from Other Cultures

Because children and non-English speaking patients from other cultures may have difficulty describing their pain verbally or rating it in terms of numerical pain assessment scales,

Principle One: Assess for Multiple Causes of Pain

extra care must be taken to ensure their pain is adequately assessed.[5] See the previous section, *Use Pain Assessment Scales*.

Children

When assessing pain in children, careful attention should be paid to the following issues:

- The child's developmental stage and its effect on the meanings of pain
- The child's developmental stage and its effect on the meaning of the child's prognosis
- The child/parent relationship
- The common occurrence of regression, i.e., increased dependency, during profound illness

Patients from Other Cultures

When assessing pain in patients from different cultures, careful attention should be paid to the following issues:

- Cultural differences in the meanings of pain
- Cultural differences in religious practices
- Cultural expectations regarding reactions to pain, i.e., stoicism or emotional expression

Patients with HIV Disease

Patients with HIV disease present special assessment challenges because, as a group, they experience unusual amounts of social, psychological, and spiritual pain resulting from conditions such as the following:

- Social isolation and blaming
- Chronic serial grief from the loss of many loved ones

In this patient population, different types of physical pain result not only from some of the drugs used to treat HIV disease but also from the disease itself. HIV disease-related conditions that cause pain include the following:

- Nerve damage pain
- Pain caused by infections such as oral candidiasis or CMV colitis[6]

Patients with HIV disease typically underreport their physical pain to physicians. Patients may rate their physical pain as 9 on a 10–point scale, but then report little pain to the physician because they are afraid their requests for pain relief will:

- Distract the physician from curative measures when they desperately want to be cured
- Label them as drug seekers

HIV patients may have a history of recreational drug use, which can complicate pain management, but that does not obviate the need for careful assessment and the prescription of adequate amounts of opioids and other analgesics.

Listen During the Assessment Process

During the assessment process, careful and attentive listening can achieve the following:

- Encourage patients to provide information that helps with the identification of multiple causes of pain
- Reassure both the patient and the family of the physician's interest in the patient's total pain
- Demonstrate the physician's confidence that something can be done to control pain

Assess For Pain Caused by Noncancer-related Physical Conditions

During the assessment process, look for pain caused by pre-existing and noncancer-related conditions such as:

Arthritis: Consider the use of nonsteroidal anti-inflammatory drugs (NSAIDs) and other appropriate therapies.

Constipation: Consider the use of laxatives and other appropriate therapies. See *Anticipate Problems with Opioid Treatment* (page 32).

Decubiti: Consider regular turning, special mattresses, and other appropriate treatments. If pain interferes with movement, prescribe analgesics prior to turning.

Migraine Headaches: Consider the use of antidepressants, ergot derivatives, and other appropriate therapies.

Muscle Strain: Consider massage, heating pads, relaxants, and other appropriate therapies.

Oral Thrush: Consider the use of topical or systemic antifungals.

Surgery and Injuries: Consider the use of physical therapy, opioids, and other appropriate analgesics.

Principle One: *Assess for Multiple Causes of Pain*

Assess for Cancer-related Physical Pain

An effective assessment depends on the physician's ability to differentiate cancer-related pains so type-specific treatments can be initiated. Because patients frequently experience several different types of cancer-related pain concurrently, the adjectives they use can help identify each type of pain.

Bone Pain and Soft Tissue Pain

Bone pain intensifies on movement and is often tender to palpation. As with soft tissue pain, it is often described as "tender" or "deep and aching." It is responsive to opioids, but also may require an adjuvant drug. See *Use Adjuvant Drugs When Necessary* (page 38). Soft tissue pain usually responds well to opioid treatment.

Neuropathic or Nerve Damage Pain

This type of pain is often described as "shooting," "burning," "stabbing," or "scalding," and usually follows the distribution of a sensory nerve. It may present with allodynia—pain from light touch or mild pressure. It does not respond completely to opioids. Adjuvant drugs are usually necessary.

Raised Intracranial Pressure Pain

This type of pain is often described as generalized or posterior head pain and is usually accompanied by nausea. It may not respond completely to opioids and often requires the use of adjuvant drugs.

Visceral pain or colic pain

These pains may be described as "spasms" or "cramping." They may respond completely to opioids, but adjuvant drugs can be very helpful in some cases.

Assess for Nonphysical Causes of Pain

Pain is not simply a matter of an impulse traveling along a nerve; it is much more. Total pain—a term used to describe the all-encompassing pain experienced by terminally ill patients—is a combination of four different types of pain. Because each component of total pain interacts with the others, hospice/palliative care can be effective only if it addresses all four of the following components of total pain:

- Physical pain
- Emotional pain, including anxiety, depression, and other types of psychological distress
- Social pain, including isolation and abandonment
- Spiritual pain, including a sometimes agonizing search for meaning and purpose

Terminally ill patients frequently harbor death-related anxieties and fears but may be reluctant to discuss them for fear their thoughts and feelings might be considered strange or abnormal. Physicians should inquire carefully about the presence of psychological, social, and spiritual pain and help normalize their presence by providing reassurance that most patients have similar concerns. With nonjudgmental listening and a caring presence, physicians can provide emotional support that sometimes is more important than additional tests or medications.

During the assessment process, estimating the severity of nonphysical pain is as important as rating the severity of cancer-related physical pain. Nonjudgmental listening and education often can alleviate mild nonphysical pain, but the presence of moderate to severe nonphysical pain calls for more potent interventions such as the involvement of counselors, social workers, or chaplains and the addition of pharmacological therapies when anxiety or depression interfere with quality of life.

Table 1

	Four Components of Total PAIN
P	**Physical** problems, often multiple, must be specifically diagnosed and treated.[7]
A	**Anxiety,** anger, and depression are critical components of pain that must be addressed by the physician in conjunction with other health care professionals.
I	**Interpersonal** problems, including loneliness, financial stress, and family tensions, are often interwoven in the fabric of a patient's symptoms.
N	**Non-acceptance** of approaching death, a sense of hopelessness, and a desperate search for meaning in life can cause severe suffering unrelieved by medications.

Open-ended Assessment Questions

It is important to use open-ended questions to assess for the presence of nonphysical pain. Examples of open-ended questions that may elicit information about psychosocial and spiritual pain include the following:

- When people become seriously ill, they usually find themselves wondering why it happened to them. When you wonder about it, what comes to mind?
- When you think about the next few weeks or months, what are some of the concerns that come to your mind first? What things concern you more than others?
- When you think back over the years, what are some of your happiest times? Saddest?
- What has given you strength in the past? What gives you strength now? What do you wish could happen to give you more strength?
- How has this illness affected you emotionally? What has been particularly difficult? Has anything been more (less) difficult than you thought it might be?
- How is your family coping with this illness? Can you tell me something about what is going on with them? What are some of your concerns about your family?

Clinical Situation Illustrating the Assessment of Multiple Causes of Pain

Clinical Situation: William and Evelyn G.

William G. is a 63-year-old male veteran who was diagnosed one year ago with adenocarcinoma of the lung, metastatic to the other lung. He has undergone radiation therapy and one dose of chemotherapy that caused such severe nausea and vomiting he refused further treatment. He was referred for hospice care.

During the hospice physician's home assessment visit in William and Evelyn's very modest home, William complains of severe pain that does not respond to the oral 4 mg hydromorphone (Dilaudid) tablets prescribed by his attending physician every 4 hours as needed for pain. During the interview William moans and reports all-over, aching pain but is unable to rate it on a numerical scale. He is obviously miserable.

Question One

What is the most appropriate course of action to take now?

[A] Prescribe a higher dose of hydromorphone (Dilaudid).

[B] Add an adjuvant drug.

[C] Order a set of electrolytes and blood urea nitrogen.

[D] Transfer William to the hospital for IV morphine.

[E] Perform a complete history and physical.

Correct Response and Analysis

The correct response is E. A thorough history and physical is required to adequately assess multiple causes of pain. In this case, more information is needed about the causes of William's pain before any decisions are made about medication orders or tests. The simple maneuver of completing a history and physical is much more likely to be productive and will cause the patient the least amount of pain and expense. Blood chemistries and counts will not provide the essential information needed.

Principle One: *Assess for Multiple Causes of Pain*

The Case Continues: History and Physical Exam

The physician's first questions relate to the location of William's pain. When asked to point to all the places where he hurts, William eventually indicates his chest, stomach, and back. William clearly has tenderness on his chest wall and sacrum and is experiencing cramping discomfort in the lower abdomen.

The history further reveals that William is bed-bound most of the time and needs assistance with turning. When discussing his medication, William says he had been taking Tylenol #3 but it did not control the pain so his physician prescribed hydromorphone (Dilaudid). He reports falling asleep after taking 4 mg of hydromorphone (Dilaudid) and then feeling somewhat drowsy and confused when he awakens. Although he is experiencing persistent pain, he takes only 1 hydromorphone (Dilaudid) tablet every other day because he wants to remain awake. The history also reveals that William has not had a bowel movement in 4 days. His wife is arthritic and is having increasing difficulty caring for William.

The physical exam reveals a cachectic male who appears older than his stated age. The exam is remarkable for decreased breath sounds on both sides of his chest, tenderness to the left side of the chest wall near the radiation therapy skin changes, and mild lower abdominal distention consistent with constipation. The rectal exam reveals a soft fecal impaction but no masses. He has a Stage II decubitus on his sacrum and severe muscle wasting.

Question Two

The four most likely causes of William's pain are:

[A] Neuropathic pain

[B] Bony/soft tissue pain from lung cancer

[C] Pain from a decubitus ulcer

[D] Pain from constipation

[E] Pain from inadequate analgesia (incorrect dose and poor compliance)

Correct Response and Analysis

The correct responses are B, C, D, and E. William describes his pain as "all over and aching" and has chest-wall tenderness underneath the radiation therapy marks, all of which indicate the presence of bone/soft tissue pain resulting from bone and tissue involvement. William has a bedsore consistent with decreased mobility and lack of turning, he describes lower abdominal cramping consistent with not having had a bowel movement in 4 days, and he is noncompliant with analgesia orders because the hydromorphone (Dilaudid) causes drowsiness and he wants to stay awake.

A is incorrect. Neuropathic pain appears to be an unlikely source of pain because the patient does not describe the stinging, burning, radiating pain along nerve distribution routes that characterizes such pain.

The Case Continues: Nonphysical Causes of Pain

Further discussion with William reveals that he is extremely angry and depressed about being fired from his job immediately after being diagnosed with cancer. He is worried that the financial pressures created by his illness will result in the loss of their home, leaving his wife with no place to live. Evelyn is fearful about how she is going to manage now that William can no longer provide financial support.

Question Three

What are two additional causes of William's pain?

[A] Emotional /psychological pain
[B] Social pain
[C] Spiritual pain

Correct Response and Analysis

The correct responses are A and B. In this situation William expresses emotional pain, evidenced by his anger and depression, and social pain as evidenced by his worry about financial matters.

Principle One: *Assess for Multiple Causes of Pain*

Question Four

How might William's social and emotional pain affect the course of his illness?

[A] They are irrelevant to the management of William's care.

[B] They are likely to complicate medication compliance.

[C] They are likely to exacerbate physical pain.

[D] They are likely to prevent William from acceptance of his approaching death.

Correct Response and Analysis

The correct answers are B, C, and D. Concerns about the cost of purchasing medicines may interfere with William's compliance with medication orders. Both emotional and social pain create stress and anxiety that can exacerbate physical pain and interfere with the acceptance of approaching death. William is unlikely to rest comfortably until his financial problems are addressed.

(This clinical situation continues on page 45)

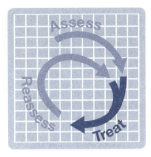

Principle Two

Treat Each Type of Pain

- Introduction to Treatment

- Treat Pain Caused by Noncancer-related Physical Conditions

- Treat Cancer-related Physical Pain
    - Dispel Misconceptions About Morphine
    - Remember Categories of Opioid Responsiveness
    - Use Effective Opioid Dosing
    - Anticipate Problems with Opioid Treatment
    - Use Adjuvant Drugs When Necessary
    - Use Nonpharmacological Methods When Appropriate
    - Avoid Placebos

- Treat Nonphysical Causes of Pain
    - Suffering: A Definition
    - Physician As Healer

- Continuing Clinical Situation Illustrating the Treatment of Multiple Causes of Pain

Principle Two: *Treat Each Type of Pain*

Introduction to Treatment

Effective treatment of total pain depends on thorough assessments and specific interventions designed to relieve each type of pain. Most physical pain can be managed with relatively simple techniques, but effective control requires individualized treatment and medication dosages adequate to control the intensity of pain being experienced.

In most cases, the practitioner can control pain adequately by:

- Following the World Health Organization's process for titrating oral pharmacological therapy
- Correctly calculating oral and injectable morphine equivalents
- Using effective starting doses and titrating upward as needed.
- Using appropriate adjuvant drugs to treat each type of pain
- Anticipating problems with treatment such as constipation or sedation
- Incorporating nonpharmacological methods such as distraction and relaxation

Treating severe nonphysical pain and suffering presents a more challenging task for most physicians, but the following can be helpful:

- Involving all members of the interdisciplinary team, including the chaplain, social worker, and other counselors with expertise in grief-related issues
- Using pharmacological therapy to treat disabling anxiety and depression
- Offering supportive and caring presence while the patient searches for renewed hope, purpose, and meaning

Treat Pain Caused by Noncancer-related Physical Conditions

Because descriptions of appropriate treatments for noncancer-related sources of pain such as arthritis, decubiti, migraine headaches, muscle strain, and oral thrush are widely available elsewhere, they are not included in this UNIPAC (other than the brief suggestions on page 11). For more information on the treatment of constipation, see *Anticipate Problems with Opioid Treatment* (page 32).

Treat Cancer-related Physical Pain

Dispel Misconceptions About Morphine

Many physicians are reluctant to prescribe morphine due to misconceptions about its effects. Nurses may be reluctant to administer (and patients may be reluctant to use) morphine or other opioids for many of the same reasons. Some of the most common misconceptions about morphine and other opioids include the following[8]:

Morphine ≠ respiratory depression

Clinically significant respiratory depression is extremely rare in patients who are receiving optimal doses of morphine. When morphine is carefully titrated, it is a safe analgesic, even for patients with respiratory disease. Morphine has been shown to be safe and effective for treating the dyspnea associated with cancer[9,10] and chronic obstructive pulmonary disease.[11]

Due to concerns about respiratory depression, some physicians recommend the use of naloxone whenever respirations drop below 12 per minute; however, the use of naloxone is inappropriate in most of these cases. Many terminally ill patients experience respirations of 6-12 per minute when asleep or awake. Clinically significant respiratory depression may be suspected when both the patient's level of consciousness and respirations drop concomitantly, with respirations reaching <6/minute; however, as long as the patient is arousable and/or breathing >6/minute, naloxone should not be administered. Simple dosage reduction is usually adequate if the patient is truly over medicated. See *Opioid Overdose* (page 37).

When terminally ill patients who have been on stable doses of opioids for several days develop the symptoms listed below, the normal dying process has begun. The appropriate action is to talk with the patient's family about the dying process, ***not*** to order naloxone.

A common symptom of dying is decreased or erratic respirations (some terminally ill patients die in a hyperventilatory state as a result of sepsis, acidosis, or respiratory muscle fatigue), in conjunction with:

- Extreme weakness
- Decreased alertness, usually with confusion
- Cool extremities

Morphine ≠ addiction

Physical dependence (withdrawal symptoms on abrupt discontinuation) is an expected result of long-term opioid treatment, but it should not be confused with psychological addiction.[1] Psychological addiction (a craving that results in drug-seeking behavior) is an extremely rare occurrence when morphine is administered to cancer patients in regularly scheduled and individually titrated doses.[12] When radiation or other treatments eliminate pain, the vast majority of patients can then be tapered off opioids without withdrawal symptoms. Many patients who fear addiction are reassured by the fact that they can be tapered off opioids easily *if* their pain can be relieved by treatments such as radiation.

Morphine ≠ rapid tolerance

Due to concerns about opioid tolerance, many physicians save the use of opioids for the very end of a patient's life, but the presence of unrelieved pain, not the patient's prognosis, should determine when opioids are used. Clinically significant tolerance is unusual because the therapeutic range of opioids is very wide. After an effective baseline dose is established, dose requirements usually plateau until disease progression occurs, at which time increased doses are necessary to control increased levels of pain.

Morphine ≠ imminent death

Many patients and family members are reluctant to use opioids because they equate the use of opioids with imminent death. By refusing opioids, patients and family members think they can magically forestall death. Due to concerns about tolerance and addiction, physicians may inadvertently reinforce this misconception and cause increased suffering when they withhold opioids until the very end of the patient's life. Because pain is both psychologically and physically destructive, unrelieved pain may actually shorten survival time.

Morphine ≠ narrow effective dose range

Morphine has a very wide effective dose range. Two milligrams of oral morphine every 4 hours may be an effective dose for some patients, while others may require more than 300 mg every 4 hours. When morphine is carefully titrated to control pain in terminally ill patients, there is no one maximal dose.

Morphine ≠ ineffective by mouth

Oral morphine is a very effective analgesic for most patients until death is imminent and swallowing becomes difficult. When prescribing oral morphine, physicians need to remember it is one-third (1/3) as potent as parenteral morphine. Effective doses must be ordered.

Morphine ≠ nausea

Nausea is a common physiologic response to morphine and may be experienced by up to 30% of patients when therapy is first begun. When patients have experienced bouts of nausea associated with morphine use, they may believe they are allergic to morphine, but that is almost never the case. The appropriate action is to prescribe a lower starting dose of morphine and to order an antiemetic, which can often be withdrawn after several days or weeks with no return of the nausea. Prescribing a different strong opioid such as oxycodone or hydromorphone is another good alternative. Patients who have been taking regular doses of other opioids such as oxycodone or hydrocodone rarely experience nausea when they are switched to morphine. See *Anticipate Problems with Opioid Treatment* (page 32).

Morphine ≠ euphoria

Morphine does not cause euphoria in terminally ill patients; however, a patient's mood may improve if relief from pain provides a good night's sleep. In hospice/palliative care, boosts in mood are more likely to be caused by steroids, dronabinol (Marinol), and methylphenidate (Ritalin).

Remember Categories of Opioid Responsiveness

From a pharmacological point of view, cancer-related pain can be divided into four treatment categories, each of which describes a specific pain's responsiveness to opioid therapy. In many cases, the correct dose of oral morphine provides effective relief from pain without the use of an adjuvant drug.

1. Opioid responsive pain

Soft tissue pain usually responds well to opioid analgesics such as morphine. See *Use Effective Opioid Dosing* (page 25).

2. Pain that is partially responsive to opioids

Bone pain may be only partially responsive to opioids, and it often requires a combination of morphine and an NSAID or another adjuvant. Some neuropathic (nerve damage) pains may respond partially to high-dose opioids, but this kind of pain usually requires an adjuvant drug such as an antidepressant or an anticonvulsant. Visceral pain may respond to an opioid, but it usually requires an anticholinergic. See *Use Effective Opioid Dosing* (page 25) and *Use Adjuvant Drugs When Necessary* (page 38).

3. Pain that is opioid responsive, but the use of opioids is inappropriate

Prescribing opioids to control pain caused by constipation, bladder distension, or a Stage I decubitis ulcer is an example of an inappropriate use of opioids. Pains such as these should be treated with other, specific measures. For more information on constipation, see *Anticipate Problems with Opioid Treatment* (page 32).

4. Opioid nonresponsive pain

Pains such as some neuropathic pains and muscle spasm pain may not respond completely to opioid analgesia regardless of dose; other drugs must be used. Neuropathic pain is caused by nerve destruction and is characteristically dermatomal in distribution.[13] Patients usually describe pure neuropathic pain as burning or scalding, and antidepressants are an appropriate first-line treatment. When neuropathic pain is described as shooting, stabbing pain that radiates from the plexus or spinal root, it should be treated with an anticonvulsant. Often, both drugs are required.

Muscle spasm pain may not respond to morphine and should be treated with local heat and massage, relaxation therapy, some tranquilizers such as diazepam, trigger point injections of a local anesthetic, and/or a corticosteroid.

For additional information on the treatment of each type of cancer-related pain, see *Use Effective Opioid Dosing* (page 25) and *Use Adjuvant Drugs When Necessary* (page 38).

Use Effective Opioid Dosing

When nonopioid analgesics such as acetaminophen or NSAIDs no longer control pain, the appropriate action usually is to prescribe opioids. Opioids are the safest and most effective agents for most types of cancer-related pain; however, they are effective only when prescribed in effective doses.

Prescribing Analgesics

The World Health Organization (WHO) recommends a simple and effective **three-step** process, or ladder, for titrating pharmacologic therapy that provides effective pain relief for more than 90% of patients with cancer.[1]

- **Step One**—The first step of the ladder is to use acetaminophen, aspirin, or other NSAIDs to relieve mild to moderate pain.

- **Step Two**—When pain persists or increases, the second step is to *add* an opioid such as codeine or hydrocodone to the NSAID. At this second step, fixed-dose combinations of an opioid with acetaminophen or aspirin are often used because combining the drugs provides additive analgesia. When higher doses of codeine or hydrocodone are needed, separate-dosage forms of the opioid and nonopioid are used to avoid the adverse side effects of high-dose acetaminophen and other NSAIDs. When the second step is initiated, medications for persistent pain are administered on an *around-the-clock* basis with additional "as-needed" booster doses to control breakthrough pain.

- **Step Three**—The third step of the ladder is to replace a weak opioid such as codeine or hydrocodone with a more potent opioid such as morphine or hydromorphone. The third step is initiated when, despite treatment with a weaker opioid, pain persists or increases. Patients who are experiencing moderate to severe pain when first seen by the clinician are usually started at the second or third step of the ladder.[1]

NOTE—Adjuvant drugs may be used at any step to: (1) enhance analgesia, (2) treat concurrent symptoms that exacerbate pain, and (3) provide independent analgesia for specific types of pain. Adjuvant drugs, or co-analgesics, are medications that have analgesic properties for specific types of pain even though they are not usually thought of as pain relievers. Examples of adjuvant drugs include antidepressants used to alleviate neuropathic pain and anticholinergics used to help control visceral pain. See *Use Adjuvant Drugs when Necessary* (page 38).

Principle Two: *Treat Each Type of Pain*

Table 2

Oral Morphine Equivalents

Oral Morphine Equivalent	Easiest to Swallow	Also Useful	Notes
1-2 mg	codeine soluble tablet* 30 mg	APAP** + Codeine 30 mg (Tylenol #3)	• Codeine with APAP and hydrocodone are the **only** drugs on this list that **do not require a triplicate prescription** (in states that require them).
	oxycodone elixir 1cc (5 mg/5 cc)	hydrocodone 5 mg (Hycodan)	
5 mg	oxycodone elixir 5 cc (5 mg/5 cc)	oxycodone 5 mg + APAP 325 mg (Percocet)	• Oxycodone is rarely nauseating.
	morphine dissolve 10 mg soluble tablet in 2 cc of water and give 1cc	oxycodone 5 mg + APAP 500 mg (Tylox)	• Avoid hepatic APAP toxicity by limiting APAP dose to <1000 mg (3 Percocet or 2 Tylox) every 4 hrs.
10 mg	morphine 10 mg soluble tablet	morphine 10 mg/ 5cc syrup	• Syrup is too dilute for use at higher doses.
	hydromorphone (Dilaudid) 2.5 mg tablets	morphine 30 mg slow-release tabs, 1 q 12 hrs. (MS Contin 30 mg or Oramorph SR 30 mg)	• Slow-release tablets are not useful for booster doses.
15 mg (= 5 mg IM morphine)	morphine 15 mg soluble tablet	morphine 30 mg slow-release tabs, 1 q 8 hrs. (MS Contin 30 mg or Oramorph SR 30 mg)	• Do not crush slow-release tablets.
20 mg	hydromorphone (Dilaudid) 5 mg	morphine 20 mg/cc solution 1 ml (Roxanol)	• Concentrated liquids require careful measuring.
30 mg (=10 mg IM morphine)	morphine 30 mg soluble tablet	Higher doses from multiples of the above. (Oramorph MS Contin) 60 mg 1 tab every 8 hrs.	* Soluble tablets are immediate-release with rapid dissolution times. ** APAP = acetaminophen

The five basic concepts of the WHO ladder for controlling pain are:

(1) By the mouth
(2) By the clock
(3) By the ladder
(4) For the individual
(5) With attention to detail

Oral Morphine Equivalents

When a stronger opioid or a different formulation is needed, the easiest way to calculate the required potency is to first convert the opioid to its oral morphine equivalent. Using this method, a physician can compare potencies and order effective doses of medication. Table 2 illustrates oral morphine equivalents.

Examples:

- A patient who is taking 2 oxycodone 5 mg plus acetaminophen (Percocet) tablets obtains good pain relief but begins to have difficulty swallowing. As shown in Table 2, 5 mg of oxycodone has the same potency as 5 mg of oral morphine. Because the patient's pain is relieved for 4 hours with 10 mg of oxycodone, an order for an equivalent amount of oral morphine—10 mg of oral morphine every 4 hours—should continue to provide effective pain relief.

- When difficulty with swallowing occurs, soluble tablets may be an alternative. They dissolve in water (or in the mouth) in about 30 seconds and are inexpensive, easy to count, and can be taken orally or sublingually. An example is Solutab, a very small soluble tablet made by Eli Lilly. For more information on the use of soluble tablets, concentrated solutions, and rectal preparations, see *Reassess Need for Alternative Routes of Drug Administration* (page 54).

- If 2 tablets of codeine 30 mg or 2 hydrocodone 5 mg tablets, are not providing good pain relief for 4 hours, prescribe 1 oxycodone 5 mg tablet every 4 hours. When 2 oxycodone 5 mg tablets no longer provide 4 hours of pain relief, prescribe 15 mg of oral morphine every 4 hours.

Injectable Morphine Equivalents

When patients can no longer swallow oral medications, continuous subcutaneous infusion (SC) or intravenous (IV) delivery are effective alternative routes of medication administration and may be required. Intramuscular injections are painful and usually unnecessary. To calculate effective parenteral doses, begin with oral morphine equivalents.

The following method is recommended for converting oral morphine to an equivalent SC dose of morphine:

(1) Calculate the patient's total daily requirement of oral morphine.

(2) Divide that dose by 3 to determine the patient's total daily requirement of subcutaneous morphine.

The following method is recommended for converting oral morphine to an equivalent dose of SC hydromorphone (Dilaudid):

(1) Calculate the patient's total daily requirement of oral morphine.

(2) Divide that dose by 20 to determine the patient's total daily dose of SC hydromorphone (Dilaudid).

NOTE—When converting oral hydromorphone to SC hydromorphone, divide the oral dose by 5.

For more information about subcutaneous delivery, see *Reassess Need for Alternative Routes of Drug Administration* (page 54).

Table 3

Conversion of Oral Opioid Doses to Parenteral Doses

Drug	PO	SC or IV
Morphine	20 mg → divide by 3 → ~7 mg	
	divide by 20 ↘	
Hydromorphone	5 mg → divide by 5 → 1 mg	

Notes:
(1) Observe the patient carefully when changing opioids; due to limited cross-tolerance between opioids, some patients will require smaller doses when opioids are changed.
(2) To determine an hourly SC dose, divide the patient's total daily SC dose by 24.

Opioid Starting Doses

The appropriate starting dose of morphine depends on the following:

- Patient's age, body weight, and degree of cachexia
- Total daily dose of previous analgesics
- Frequency and severity of pain

When initiating opioid therapy, the best policy is to begin with a low dose (see Table 4) and then rapidly titrate upward until relief is achieved. Morphine doses can be increased by 30% to 100% or more each day as needed until pain is relieved. Except for slow-release tablets or patches, the opioid should be prescribed every 4 hours on a regular schedule; however, a double dose at bedtime usually lasts 8 hours and allows uninterrupted sleep. Instruct the patient to take a booster dose when breakthrough pain occurs. See *Opioid Titration* (page 31).

When circumstances make it difficult to determine an appropriate opioid dose, avoid medication delivery systems that cannot be rapidly adjusted, for example sustained-release or transdermal preparations. Until an effective opioid baseline dose has been established, it is important to use medications that can be rapidly and accurately titrated.

Special Populations

Children, the frail elderly, and patients with HIV disease present special pain-management challenges that often result in gross under treatment of their pain. Careful assessments and effective doses of medication are particularly important with these populations.

Infants and Children

The high-dose chemotherapy agents used to treat cancer in infants and children often result in treatment-related conditions such as neuropathies, mouth ulcers, and joint pain that may cause more pain than the disease itself, particularly in the case of leukemia. When caring for children, adequately assessing and treating treatment-related sources of pain often is as important as adequately controlling cancer-related pain.

When treating opioid-responsive pain in children, see Table 5. Start with the recommended doses (usually of codeine or hydrocodone) and rapidly titrate to effect, which often results in doses several times larger than the starting dose.

Table 4

Starting Doses for Opioid-naive Patients

• Infant or child (with mild pain and great concern about side effects)	• Child with moderate to severe pain, or • Adult <60 kg, or • Elderly patient, or • Adult with mild pain	• Adult > 60 kg (with moderate to severe pain and fear that pain will never be relieved)
Start with: < 2 mg oral morphine equivalent every 4 hours (see Table 5)	**Start with:** 2-5 mg oral morphine equivalent every 4 hours, e.g. 1/2-1 oxycodone and acetaminophen (Percocet) q 4 hrs	**Start with:** 5-10 mg oral morphine equivalent every 4 hours, e.g. 1/2-1 morphine 10 mg soluble tablet q 4 hrs

Frail Elderly

When treating frail elderly patients, begin with half of the usual adult opioid dose and rapidly titrate the dose to effect.

Patients with HIV Disease

Because patients with HIV disease may have contracted their disease from drug abuse-related behavior, physicians frequently are reticent to prescribe opioids because of concerns about drug misuse; however, such concerns can result in gross under treatment of HIV patients who are experiencing very high levels of pain. While it is easy to confuse a patient's drug-seeking request forstronger doses of medication with a request for relief from uncontrolled pain, careful assessment can help establish reliable reports of pain and provide physician reassurance that appropriate opioid doses are being prescribed. See *Assess for Multiple Causes of Pain* (page 8).

When treating pain in this patient population, remember:

- It is easy to confuse requests for drugs that result from under treatment of pain with requests related to the drug-seeking behavior of addiction.

- Careful assessments can help provide reliable reports of pain.

- Treating pain in the drug-abusing population presents special challenges, but it can be done.[14]

- Pain frequently is under treated in the HIV population.

- Physicians can set medication limits while making sure adequate doses are prescribed.

- Information is available on controlling pain in the drug-abusing patient.[15]

Table 5

Initial Oral Opioid Doses for Children

< 50 kilograms and > 6 months

0.5-1 mg/kg every 3-4 hours of codeine

0.2 mg/kg every 3-4 hours of hydrocodone or oxycodone

0.3 mg/kg every 3-4 hours of morphine

0.06 mg/kg every 3-4 hours of hydromorphone

< 6 Months

Begin with 1/4 to 1/3 of the above doses and rapidly titrate to effect.

- Patients with histories of drug abuse also experience high levels of disease-related pain and should be treated.

Opioid Titration

Because cancer pain usually increases over time, titrating opioids to provide effective individualized doses is an important pain management technique that is used daily in hospice/palliative care settings. There is no ceiling or maximal recommended opioid dose; large doses of morphine, e.g., several hundred mg every 4 hours, may be needed to relieve severe pain.

During the titration process, the physician must remember that immediate-release morphine is a 4-hour drug that reaches its peak effect in approximately 2 hours when delivered orally, and in about 10-20 minutes when delivered subcutaneously. When pain is not relieved within peak times of a higher dose, an additional dose should be given. During the titration process, no ceiling exists on the number of times a dose may be titrated. Over a 24-hour period, some patients may require more than a 100% increase over their initial daily baseline dose. See Table 6 and *Breakthrough Pain* (page 32).

NOTE—During the entire titration process, continuing reassessment is needed to identify the presence of the following:

- Pain that does not respond to opioids that must be treated with adjuvant drugs or other specific remedies. See (page 38).

- Nonphysical pain that must be treated with compassionate listening and involvement of other members of the interdisciplinary team. See *UNIPAC Two: Psychological, Spiritual and Physiological Aspects of Dying and Bereavement.*

Table 6
Titration Increments for Opioid Dosing*

Baseline 4-hour Dose	Titration Increment (~1/2 of 4-hour dose)
1-10 mg	1-5 mg
10-20 mg 5-10 mg	
20-30 mg 10-15 mg	
40-50 mg	20-25 mg
100 mg	30-50 mg
200 mg	50-100 mg
500 mg	100-250 mg
1,000 mg	250-500 mg

*These increment doses are also appropriate for use as "booster doses." See *Breakthrough Pain* (below).

Breakthrough Pain

Because breakthrough pain is a common problem for many patients, additional opioid doses should be prescribed on an as-needed basis. These additional opioid doses (referred to as "booster" doses because they boost the analgesic level) should be approximately 1/2 the regular 4-hour opioid dose, or about 10% of the 24-hour dose. Regular use of booster doses (more than 3-4 times daily) may signal the need for an increase in the baseline dose and/or the need for a co-analgesic. See Table 6 for examples of appropriate booster doses.

Drugs and Routes to Avoid in Hospice/Palliative Care

Table 7 describes drugs and medication delivery routes that should be avoided in hospice/palliative care settings.

Anticipate Problems with Opioid Treatment

Patient Compliance

In most cases, patient compliance improves when physicians take time to listen carefully to patient/family concerns and provide further education about opioid use and treatable side effects. Patient and family concerns about opioid use are often based on misconceptions. Compliance problems also arise from conditions such as swallowing difficulties, concerns about opioid-related constipation, and lack of patient access to expensive medications.

Table 7

Drugs and Routes to Avoid in Hospice/Palliative Care	
Meperidine (Demerol)	Very low potency. Toxic metabolite accumulation.
Pentazocine (Talwin)	No more potent than codeine. High incidence of hallucinations and agitation (30% in cancer patients). Inhibits analgesia of morphine.
Methadone (Dolophine)	Extremely long half life (48-72 hours) and short duration of analgesia (6-8 hours) make dose titration difficult in severely ill patients. Can be effective when used by experienced practitioners if patients develop tolerance or allergy to morphine and hydromorphine.
IM Injections	Morphine 30 mg PO is as potent as 10 mg IM/SC. Avoid the pain and expense of injections with PO or SL morphine. If patient cannot tolerate anything PO, start a SC infusion or give slow-release morphine tablets rectally.
Opioid Suppositories	Morphine and hydromorphone suppositories are available but very few patients tolerate suppositories every 4 hours, few dose strengths are available, and SL soluble tablets or SC infusions are effective alternatives.

Adverse Side Effects

Common adverse side effects include constipation, nausea, sedation, confusion, and hallucinations. Less common side effects include urinary retention (which can result from constipation-related impactions) and myoclonic jerks.

Constipation

Most patients in hospice/palliative care settings require a maintenance laxative regimen to prevent and/or relieve constipation, a symptom commonly experienced by terminally ill patients due to the following:

- Low fluid and fiber intake
- Impaired mobility
- Complicating medical conditions, such as bowel obstructions and hemorrhoids
- Drug therapies that impair gut motility

Constipation is such a common side effect of opioid use, *nearly all* patients receiving opioid therapy should be placed on regular doses of laxatives to prevent its distressing symptoms. A combination of a softening agent and a stimulant laxative should be used, and dosages should be increased as opioid doses increase. Effective prevention requires constant vigilance and awareness of the physiological and social components of constipation.

Assessment of Constipation

On admission, each patient should be carefully assessed for constipation. The assessment should include:

- **Step One**—a detailed bowel history that includes information on:
  1. Stool frequency and consistency
  2. Previous laxative use and its effectiveness
  3. Associated problems, such as lack of privacy or long distances to the toilet
- **Step Two**—abdominal examination
- **Step Three**—rectal exam, if indicated

Impaction Removal

- **Hard impaction**—If a hard fecal impaction is found, digital removal should follow fecal softening with an oil-retention enema and perhaps premedication with diazepam or midazolam.
- **Soft impaction**—Soft impactions may respond to bisacodyl suppositories or large volume tap water or saline (phosphate) enemas.

To prevent recurrence of constipation, the removal of hard and soft impactions must be followed with a vigorous laxative protocol that includes both stool softeners and stimulant agents such as senna or bisacodyl with docusate.

Suggested Laxative Regimen

Patients with a history of constipation may wish to continue using whichever laxative has produced results in the past. Avoid bulk-forming agents such as psyllium or methylcellulose because they tend to form impactions when patients can no longer take adequate amounts of fluids.

Patients with no previous history of constipation can try the following:

- Docusate (Colace), or
- Docusate with casanthranol (Peri-Colace) or a similar gentle laxative

Most patients require individually titrated doses of potent bowel stimulants, such as the following:

- Senna (Senokot), or
- Bisacodyl (Dulcolax)

As with opioid therapy, the most effective laxative regimen for the control and prevention of constipation is one that follows a step-wise approach and is ongoing, instead of being administered on an as-needed basis.

The physician must specify the initial laxative regimen step on admission orders (e.g. senna 5 mg PO BID) and specify that an ongoing laxative regimen must be instituted. If the patient has not had a bowel movement in 2 days, the laxative dose should be increased to the

Table 8

An Effective Step-wise Laxative Regimen

Step	Medication	Dose
(1)	Docusate (100 mg)	1 cap BID
(2)	Senna (Senokot) or bisacodyl (Dulcolax)	1 tab QD
(3)	Senna or bisacodyl	1 tab BID
(4)	Senna or bisacodyl	2 tabs BID
(5)	Senna or bisacodyl	3 tabs BID
(6)	Senna **plus** sorbitol	4 tabs BID 15 cc BID
(7)	Senna **plus** sorbitol	to 4 tabs BID 30 cc BID
(8)	Senna **plus** sorbitol	4 tabs BID 30 cc TID-QID

Note: One generic senna tablet 187 mg ~ senna extract 5 mg (Senokot)

next level. If the patient has not had a bowel movement in 3 days, one of the following treatments is given once or twice daily until results are obtained:

- Digital disimpaction followed by 2 bisacodyl suppositories OR
- Sodium phosphate 30 cc PO repeated in 2 hours if needed OR
- Mineral oil or soapsuds enema

After successful treatment, the patient should resume the step-wise regimen at the level at which the above treatment was initiated. If none of the treatments is effective, the physician must reassess the situation and initiate appropriate therapy.

Severe Constipation

Rectal suppositories and enemas rarely are needed when a laxative regimen is conscientiously followed. However, if severe constipation develops, it should be treated vigorously. The following treatments are suggested:

- Sodium phosphate—some patients prefer a purgative dose of a saline laxative, such as sodium phosphate (Fleet Phospho-Soda), but it can cause cramping and bloating, so use 30 ml at a time PO every 2 hours.

- Bisacodyl 10 mg suppositories (1 or 2 PR) often are effective in 15 minutes to an hour.

- Soapsuds or phosphate enemas occasionally may be required.

- Higher volume enemas can increase efficacy.

- Sometimes, when nothing else works, a milk and molasses enema can be effective. Add 1 cup of powdered milk and 1 cup of molasses or corn syrup to a liter of warm water and administer rectally.

Special Situations

- **Bowel obstruction**—Patients who continue to pass some stool through their obstruction may benefit from a softening agent, such as higher-dose docusate or low-dose sorbitol. Due to the obstruction, other patients probably will vomit one or two times a day, but they can be kept comfortable on a SC infusion of an opioid and antiemetic. See *UNIPAC Four: Management of Selected Nonpain Symptoms in the Terminally Ill.*

- **Colicky abdominal pains**—Pain can be minimized with careful dose titration and/or the addition of docusate or sorbitol for stool softening. Doses of up to 300 mg of docusate tid or 30 ml of sorbitol tid are not unusual.

- **Stimulation alone is ineffective or poorly tolerated**—Osmotic agents, such as sorbitol or lactulose (Chronulac) 10 gm/15 ml (15-60 ml bid-tid), can be effective. Note: Sorbitol is less expensive, equally effective, and less nauseating than lactulose.[16]

- **Narcotic bowel syndrome**—Patients receiving opioid analgesics may develop narcotic bowel syndrome, which resembles bowel obstruction. Metoclopramide (either PO or by SC infusion) can provide relief.

Social and Psychological Aspects of Constipation

The social and psychological aspects of constipation can interfere with its treatment and prevention. Attention must be paid to:

- **Privacy needs**—A private commode with easy access is essential.

- **Acceptable caregivers**—Patients may not allow opposite-sex relatives or caretakers to give them suppositories or enemas.

- **Cost issues**—The high cost of some laxatives can interfere with compliance.

Nausea/Vomiting

When strong opioids are first prescribed, they may induce nausea and vomiting in 10% to 40% of patients. Because patients frequently believe nausea and vomiting indicate an allergic response to morphine, care should be taken to explain that such symptoms are dose-related, temporary side effects, not allergies.

When morphine is prescribed before another strong opioid such as oxycodone has been used, order an antiemetic such as prochlorperazine (Compazine) or transdermal scopolamine (Transderm Scop) for a few days to prevent nausea and vomiting. Usually, the antiemetic can be phased out after several days or weeks. Nausea or vomiting is less likely to occur if the patient has been taking regular doses of other strong opioids before starting morphine, so consider using hydrocodone or oxycodone first, if practical. For other causes and suggested treatments or nausea and vomiting, see *UNIPAC Four: Management of Selected Nonpain Symptoms in the Terminally Ill.*

Sedation/Drowsiness/Somnolence

When opioid therapy is initiated, temporary sedation frequently occurs but usually clears within 2-5 days after achieving a steady dose of effective analgesia. Although opioids directly affect the central nervous system, accumulated exhaustion and sleep deprivation caused by uncontrolled pain usually are the major contributing factors to somnolence. When pain relief is achieved, the patient finally may be able to sleep for long periods of time.

Continued drowsiness may indicate a need to decrease the opioid dose or change to a less sedating co-analgesic, but it may also be a sign of disease progression. Such sedation is **not** an indication for the use of naloxone (Narcan). If drowsiness remains troublesome, try decreasing the opioid dose and adding a nonsedating co-analgesic like a NSAID. Rotation of the opioid (i.e., morphine → hydromorphone or oxycodone) may accomplish pain relief with lower, less-sedating doses. A few patients will benefit from the addition of an amphetamine such as methylphenidate (Ritalin) 5-10 mg in the early morning and at noon.

Confusion/Hallucinations/Cognitive Impairment

Opioids may cause or aggravate confusion and hallucinations in a small number of patients, especially the elderly. If this occurs, switch to a different opioid at a lower dose, if possible. Confusion also may result from brain metastases, hepatic, renal or respiratory insufficiency, or other metabolic changes associated with advancing disease. The addition of haloperidol or a phenothiazine such as thioridazine (Mellaril) may be necessary to calm the patient. See *UNIPAC Four: The Management of Selected Nonpain Symptoms in the Terminally Ill.*

Opioid Overdose

Opioid overdose is rare when titration procedures are followed correctly; however, it can occur and should be suspected when levels of consciousness and respirations decrease concomitantly, particularly when respirations decrease to <6/minute in the presence of myoclonic twitching, constricted pupils, skeletal muscle flaccidity, and cold or clammy skin.

If the patient is drowsy and breathing slowly, stop administering opioids for a while and simply wait for the drug to wear off. Opioids can usually then be re-started at a lower dose. When administration of naloxone is necessary, **do not follow the PDR recommendations, which may cause a traumatic return of agonizing pain. Instead,** dilute 1 amp (0.4) of naloxone in 10 ml of saline and give 1 ml of this diluted mixture

(0.04 mg) IV every 5 minutes until partial reversal occurs. Repeating the process may be necessary because naloxone has a shorter half life than most opioids.

Use Adjuvant Drugs When Necessary

Several types of drugs that are not usually thought of as analgesics are referred to as co-analgesics or adjuvant drugs, because they effectively relieve certain types of pain that do not respond fully to opioid therapy.

Bone or Soft Tissue Pain—Corticosteroids/NSAIDs

Bone pain is partially responsive to opioid treatment, but it usually requires the use of anti-inflammatory drugs to provide adequate relief from its dull, aching, localized pain that worsens with movement or local pressure. If the patient has no history of low platelets, bleeding, ulcers, or renal insufficiency, an NSAID can be safe and effective, and the full antiarthritic dose is usually needed. If the patient cannot swallow, consider indomethacin (Indocin) suppositories 50 mg bid to tid or ketorolac (Toradol) 60 mg/day by SC infusion.[17]

Gastric protection may be required for elderly patients, patients with a history of ulcers, or patients using steroids. Consider using misoprostol (Cytotec) 100-200 mcg PO tid in selected situations.

When NSAIDs are contraindicated because the patient has few platelets (e.g., after chemotherapy or with extensive marrow displacement) a non acetylated salicylate such as choline magnesium trisalicylate (Trilisate) or salsalate (Disalcid) may provide some analgesia without compromising the functioning of the remaining platelets. Another option is a corticosteroid, such as dexamethasone 4 mg bid PO or SC. As with other NSAIDs, both of these alternatives may cause gastritis or peptic ulcer disease, so consider protecting the stomach with misoprostol or an H2 blocker.

Neuropathic/nerve Pain—Antidepressants/Anticonvulsants

The burning, shooting pain of neuropathic pain can be relieved with low to full doses (10-100 mg) of a tricyclic antidepressant such as amitri-ptyline (Elavil), nortriptyline (Pamelor), doxepin (Sinequan), or desipramine (Norpramin). These drugs can also help with insomnia and depression.

When neuropathic pain is characterized by shooting or stabbing pain, consider using anticonvulsants such as carbamazepine (Tegretol) or valproate (Depakene). Use full anticonvulsant dosages. In difficult cases, check for therapeutic serum levels of both the antidepressant and the anticonvulsant.

Both an antidepressant and an anticonvulsant are often required.[18] When patients cannot swallow even the liquid forms, insert doxepin capsules rectally (50 mg every 12 hours), and/or crush carbamazepine (Tegretol) tablets, put them in gelatin capsules, and give 600 mg rectally every 8-12 hours.[19] In addition to antidepressants and anticonvulsants, some antiarrhythmics such as mexiletine (Mexitil) have alleviated neuropathic pain in some patients.

Raised Intracranial Pressure—Corticosteroids

Dexamethasone 4 mg (or more) PO bid to qid is the drug of choice to relieve pain caused by raised intracranial pressure in patients whose expected length and quality of life warrant the initiation of corticosteroid therapy. When patients cannot swallow, insert a 25-gauge butterfly needle capped with an injection site into the subcutaneous tissue, secure it, and teach family members to inject the 4 mg per ml dexamethasone into the injection site 2-4 times per day. When raised intracranial pressure is associated with a rapid deterioration in the patient's mental status, a large increase in the opioid dose to control headache may be more appropriate than initiating corticosteroid therapy or giving it by injection.

Visceral Pain/Colic Pain—Anticholinergics

When cramping, coliclike abdominal pains are not due to urinary retention or fecal impaction, consider using an anticholinergic drug such as oxybutynin (Ditropan) 5-10 mg three times a day or hyoscyamine (Levsin) 0.125 mg 1-2 PO or SL every 4 hours as needed. Alert the patient to the possibility of increased constipation, dry mouth, or blurred vision. The laxative regimen may need to be increased due to worsened constipation.

If the patient cannot swallow tablets, consider sublingual hyoscyamine (Levsin SL), transdermal scopolamine (Transderm Scop), or belladonna and opioid (B&O) suppositories. Scopolamine can also be combined with an opioid and given by SC infusion.

Table 9
Suggested Adjuvant Drug Dosages

Pain Source	Pain Character	Drug Class	Examples	Notes
Bone or soft tissue	Tenderness over bone or joint, especially on movement	NSAIDs	Ibuprofen 400 mg PO q 4 hr	Inexpensive, big pills
			Sulindac (Clinoril) 200 PO mg q 12 hrs	Well tolerated, preferred in renal impairmen
			Naproxen (Naprosyn Susp) 125 mg/5cc, 15 cc PO q 8-12 hrs	Liquid preparation available
			Indomethacin (Indocin 50 mg) caps or supp. q 8 hrs	Suppository, may cause more gastritis
			Piroxicam (Feldene 20 mg) capsules, 1 PO qd	Easiest to swallow, may cause more gastritis
			Choline Mg trisalicylate (Trilisate susp) 500 mg/5cc, 15 cc q 12	Preferred in thrombocytopenia
Nerve damage or dysesthesia	Burning or scalding pain	Tricyclic anti-depressants	Amitriptyline (Elavil) 10-100 PO mg q hs	Best studied, sedating, start with low dose
			Doxepin (Sinequan) 10-100 mg PO q hs	10 mg/cc susp. available
			Trazodone (Desyrel) 25-150 mg PO q hs	+Less anticholinergic effect, 1/3 as potent as amitriptyline
	Shooting, stabbing pain	Anticonvulsants	Carbamazepine (Tegretol) 200 mg PO q 6-12 hrs Valproate (Depakote) 250 mg PO tid-qid	Both are absorbed from rectum
Visceral spasms	Colic, cramping abdominal pain, bladder spasms	Anticholinergics	Scopolamine (Transderm Scop) 1-2 patches q 3d	Scopolamine may also be mixed with narcotic in SC infusion 0.8-2.4 mg/d
			Hyoscyamine (Levsin) 0.125 mg PO or SL q 4-8 hrs	Capsules, SL tabs, or liquid
			Oxybutynin (Ditropan) 5-10 mg PO q 8 hrs	Tablets or liquid

Use Nonpharmacological Methods When Appropriate

In hospice/palliative care settings, nonpharmacologic methods of pain control are generally appropriate for use as adjunct therapies to pharmacologic treatment rather than as stand-alone treatments. The following methods can be invaluable for improving quality of life and enhancing the efficacy of drug therapy:

- Distraction—music, art, movies, reading, books on tape
- Guided imagery or hypnosis
- Progressive relaxation
- Meditation
- Massage therapy
- TENS units or acupuncture

Avoid Placebos

When pain continues to occur in the absence of clinical findings, adequate treatment of pain requires dedication, persistence, and a willingness to consider many treatment modalities. In hospice/palliative care settings, the use of placebos to control pain is prohibited by the principles of patient autonomy and informed consent, as well as by the hospice/palliative care commitment to a patient's inclusion as a member of the health care team.

Treat Nonphysical Causes of Pain

Emotional, spiritual, and social pain may be caused by conditions such as the following:

- Anxiety
- Depression
- Isolation and loneliness
- Fear
- Financial concerns
- Loss of faith
- Loss of meaning

In hospice/palliative care settings and in this UNIPAC, total pain is described as a combination of the patient's physical, social, emotional, and spiritual pain. Although this model of total pain is helpful for the purposes of emphasizing the multifaceted nature of pain, it has the unfortunate effect of reinforcing the dichotomous view of pain as being either physical or nonphysical—a view that tends to diminish the patient's suffering and relegate physicians to the role of mechanical technicians whose only purpose is the manipulation of dosages and dials.

Instead, the concept of pain must be enlarged to include physical distress **and** suffering, which are phenomenologically distinct. A person may be in severe physical pain but not be suffering because the pain is explainable and has meaning, for instance the pain of childbirth or kidney stones. However, when the source of pain is unknown and when it is chronic, overwhelming, and without meaning, it generally results in suffering.[20]

Suffering: A Definition

Suffering can be defined as "the state of severe distress associated with events that threaten the intactness of the person."[20] Suffering may occur as a result of symptoms such as acute pain or shortness of breath, but it extends beyond the physical. It occurs when patients perceive the impending destruction of their personhood, and it continues until the threat of disintegration has passed or until the patient's integrity can be restored in some way.[20] Patients may experience extreme suffering in the absence of physical pain.

Physician As Healer

In the process of providing relief from suffering, physicians can assume an important and enlarged role—that of healer. When cure is no longer possible, a healing physician assists with the following:

- Lending strength to patients who are suffering not only from the impending loss of all the relationships they have ever known, but also from the impending loss of all their unrealized hopes and dreams
- Reinforcing new definitions of hope as patients try to come to terms with the regrets of a lifetime
- Helping patients transcend their current physical state by assisting with the search for a broader context of meaning that includes family and community[20]

For patients and other laypersons, the relief of suffering (regardless of its source) is one of the primary goals of medicine. When, during the last days and months of life, the patient's need for healing seems to conflict with the physician's ongoing need to cure, poor communication may be the result. To assume the strength-lending role of healer, physicians must relieve the pain caused by non-cancer and cancer-related medical conditions, work closely with the interdisciplinary team, and then remain fully attentive as patients find meaning in their lives. See *UNIPAC Two: The Psychological, Spiritual and Physiological Aspects of Dying and Bereavement.*

Mild Nonphysical Pain— Social, Emotional, and Spiritual Pain

When assessment indicates the presence of mild nonphysical pain, supportive counseling, nonjudgmental listening, and education often can provide relief. However, to be effective, physicians must be able to discuss these real sources of pain with empathy and compassion.

Moderate to Severe Nonphysical Suffering

When more complicated social, emotional, and spiritual issues result in suffering, the physician should consider making referrals to other professionals, such as the patient's religious or spiritual adviser and/or a counselor or social worker with special training in issues related to terminal care.

The inclusion of pharmacologic treatment also must be considered when nonphysical pain and suffering result from depression and/or anxiety that:

- Is severe enough to interfere with the patient's ability to function

- Worsens rather than resolves with time

- Persists more than 7 days[21]

Disabling anxiety and depression are not necessary parts of the dying process; any hesitancy to treat them pharmacologically is as misguided as hesitancy to adequately treat cancer-related physical pain. There is accumulating evidence that antidepressant therapy (and therapy with other psychoactive drugs) can be very helpful in selected terminally ill patients who suffer from severe depression.[21] The hospice/palliative care philosophy mandates attempts to relieve all types of suffering. For more information on the challenging task of assessing and managing nonphysical causes of pain and treating anxiety and depression, see *UNIPAC Two: The Psychological, Spiritual and Physiological Aspects of Dying and Bereavement.*

Principle Two: *Treat Each Type of Pain*

Continuing Clinical Situation Illustrating the Treatment of Multiple Causes of Pain

(Continued from page 18)

Clinical Situation: William and Evelyn G.

During the first visit to William and Evelyn's home, the physician further explores William's reasons for not taking the hydromorphone (Dilaudid) as prescribed and discovers:

- William is concerned about drug addiction and says drowsiness and confusion are unacceptable side effects for him.
- Evelyn also is afraid of drug addiction and has been hiding the hydromorphone (Dilaudid). She wants William to stay awake so he will eat more and regain his strength.

The physician determines patient/family education is needed and explains the following:

- Taking pain medications for cancer pain does not lead to addiction; William can gradually stop taking his medication if his pain goes away completely.
- The drowsiness and confusion are occurring because he isn't taking medication of the appropriate strength.
- A different medication can be used that won't be quite as strong and won't cause as much drowsiness and confusion.
- It will be necessary to take the new medication on a regularly scheduled, 4-hour basis.
- Mild drowsiness may occur for the first day or two, but it won't be as bothersome as it has been with the hydromorphone (Dilaudid), and William's body will adjust to the new medicine after a day or two.
- William will be more awake and able to eat, and won't be in as much pain.
- Evelyn should call the hospice if William becomes so sleepy he can't be aroused to take his next dose of medicine; the dose will be reduced.
- William should take a booster dose if pain occurs but should call the hospice if he has to take booster doses more than 2 or 3 times in a 24-hour period so the baseline dose can be increased.

Principle Two: *Treat Each Type of Pain*

- The dose of the new medication will probably have to be adjusted up or down in the next few days, depending on how it works for William.
- Evelyn can call the hospice any time, day or night, if she has concerns about William's condition.
- All of them are working together to relieve William's pain.

William and Evelyn agree that mild drowsiness for a day or two is an acceptable side effect.

To determine the right starting dose of a new medication, the physician:

- Calculates that William's 4 mg dose of hydromorphone (Dilaudid) is roughly equivalent to 16 mg of an oral morphine (oral hydromorphone is about four times as potent as oral morphine). See Table 2, *Oral Morphine Equivalents* on page 26.
- Decides that 16 mg of oral morphine equivalent is more than William needs to control his pain but 1-2 mg is not adequate because the Tylenol #3 William had been taking prior to the hydromorphone (Dilaudid) did not provide relief.
- Concludes that 5 mg of an oral morphine equivalent every 4 hours is a good place to start because William is a normal-sized adult weighing more than 60 pounds with severe pain and it is important to avoid unacceptable side effects.

Question Five

At this point, which of the following medications is an appropriate choice:

[A] Oxycodone and acetaminophen (Percocet) 1 tablet every 4 hours

[B] Acetaminophen 1000 mg every 4 hours (alone)

[C] Slow-release morphine (MS Contin or Oramorph SR) 60 mg every 12 hours

[D] Slow-release morphine 15 mg twice daily

[E] Transdermal fentanyl patches (Duragesic) one 50 mcg per hour patch every 72 hours

Correct Response and Analysis

Correct answers are A or D. The preferable response is (A) oxycodone and acetaminophen (Percocet) because:

- Oxycodone 5 mg with acetaminophen (Percocet) is a cost-effective and widely available medication in this potency range (5 mg of oral morphine equivalent).

- An immediate release preparation allows more flexibility when rapid dose titration is needed to establish an effective baseline dose.

- In addition to his regular 4-hour dose, William needs medication for breakthrough pain. By prescribing oxycodone and acetaminophen (Percocet), one medication can be used for both purposes.

- The presence of acetaminophen may be helpful and William has no contraindicating symptoms; however, the acetaminophen limits the number of tablets that can be taken.

- Evelyn is available to administer the oxycodone and acetaminophen (Percocet) every 4 hours.

- Oxycodone without acetaminophen might be as effective and can be prescribed in higher doses but is not as widely available.

The second-choice response is (D) slow-release morphine 15 mg twice daily because:

- It is roughly equivalent to 5 mg of oral morphine every 4 hours.

- It is about the same dose as the oxycodone and acetaminophen (Percocet) but does not provide the added benefit of acetaminophen.

- Two medications are necessary: slow-release morphine for the baseline dose and oxycodone and acetaminophen (Percocet) for breakthrough pain. Using the fewest possible number of drugs is a goal of all medicine, in particular hospice medicine.

The Case Continues

The physician explains that: (1) William must take one 5 mg tablet every 4 hours around the clock, (2) he can take 1/2 tablet as a booster dose, and (3) at bedtime he can take 2 tablets so he doesn't have to set an alarm clock to take his 2 am dose. The physician then writes out a chart so William and Evelyn can check when he has taken his tablet at 6 am, 10 am, 2 pm, 6 pm, and 2 tablets at 10 pm.

Laxative Regimen
The physician does the following: (1) orders bisacodyl (Dulcolax) suppositories, (2) suggests William insert one suppository as soon as possible, (3) explains the medication usually works within an hour, (4) recommends using 2 suppositories if the first one is ineffective, (5) encourages the use of a suppository if a bowel movement does not occur at least every other day, and (6) asks Evelyn to call the hospice if William needs to use the suppositories regularly. The physician also prescribes Senokot S (senna with docusate) 1 tablet twice daily to prevent recurrent constipation.

Team Involvement

The physician concludes the visit by making arrangements for the hospice nurse and social worker to visit with William and Evelyn the next day to (1) make sure William is comfortable and awake, (2) reinforce what the physician has said about addiction, and (3) explore the family's financial needs and help them obtain available community assistance.

Evelyn calls the hospice at midnight the next night and reports that William is experiencing a lot of chest pain. The hospice RN confirms that (1) William has been taking one tablet of oxycodone and acetaminophen (Percocet) every 4 hours, (2) that his bowel movements are occurring regularly, and (3) that the pain has the same character and location as before, and so it is most likely chest wall pain from the lung cancer.

Question Six

At this point, which of the following is an appropriate order?

[A] Morphine solution (Roxanol) (morphine 20 mg/ml) 1 cc every 4 hours

[B] Oxycodone and acetaminophen (Percocet) 2 tablets every 4 hours

[C] Hydromorphone (Dilaudid) 1 tablet every 4 hours

[D] Slow-release morphine 15 mg every 8 hours

Correct Response and Analysis

Correct responses are either B or D. Both are equivalent to 5-10 mg of oral morphine, but (B) oxycodone and acetaminophen (Percocet) is the preferred response because, as the titration process continues, an immediate-release product allows more flexibility in dosing. However, at midnight it will be difficult to locate a new opioid, so a higher dose of whichever drug was selected in Question Five is the best answer.

Responses A and C are incorrect because the suggested doses are too strong.

The Case Continues

The hospice RN increases the oxycodone and acetaminophen (Percocet) to 2 tablets every 4 hours with a whole tablet as a booster dose. William is comfortable by morning.

A few days later, William is at home in a hospital bed and has an alternating pressure pad for his decubitus. Evelyn has been taught how to reposition him on a regular basis. The social worker has arranged for the following: (1) the utility company will waive William and Evelyn's overdue payments, (2) the Veterans Administration hospital will provide medications, and (3) procedures for obtaining disability payments have been initiated. The hospice chaplain has arranged for regular visits from William and Evelyn's pastor at their request.

On the next visit 3 days later, the nurse discovers William is getting good pain relief with 2 oxycodone and acetaminophen (Percocet) tablets but is sometimes confused and occasionally sees people on the wall. Evelyn thinks William is overmedicated.

Question Seven

At this point, what is the best choice for a medication order?

[A] Add aspirin 325 mg every 4 hours.

[B] Order an epidural catheter.

[C] Reduce oxycodone and acetaminophen (Percocet) and add naproxen (Naprosyn), 375 mg every 12 hours.

[D] Order an IV infusion pump.

[E] Add amitriptyline 50 mg at bedtime.

Correct Response and Analysis

William obtains good pain relief with 2 oxycodone and acetaminophen (Percocet) tablets, but the side effects are unacceptable. At this point the physician has two available options: (1) chose a different opioid in an attempt to reduce side effects or (2) lower the analgesia dose to decrease side effects and add an adjuvant to enhance analgesia.

The best response is C, reduce the oxycodone and acetaminophen (Percocet) to 1 tablet every 4 hours to relieve side effects and add naproxen (Naprosyn) 375 mg twice daily to control chest wall pain.

Principle Two: *Treat Each Type of Pain*

This situation illustrates the correct use of co-analgesics. When patients experience bone pain, it is not always necessary to immediately begin treatment with a co-analgesic such as naproxen (Naprosyn.) Because such drugs are more toxic than morphine or oxycodone and acetaminophen (Percocet), it is appropriate to begin treatment with morphine or oxycodone and acetaminophen (Percocet) and add naproxen (Naprosyn) only when needed.

- *(A)* is an incorrect response. Aspirin 325 mg every 4 hours would help relieve chest wall pain but is much more toxic to the stomach lining than naproxen (Naprosyn) and would not alleviate the opioid side effects.

- *(B)* is an incorrect response. An epidural catheter is invasive and expensive, and simpler maneuvers such as adding a different adjuvant have not been tried.

- *(D)* ordering an IV infusion pump is incorrect for the same reason as *(B)*.

- *(E)* is incorrect because amitriptyline may increase William's confusion.

The Case Concludes

The next day the RN reports that William's pain is moderately well controlled, but he is taking booster doses three times a day. The physician increases the naproxen (Naprosyn) to 375 mg three times a day with good relief of chest wall pain and no return of the confusion.

After several weeks William's pain begins to increase, so he is switched to oral morphine 15 mg every 4 hours with good pain control and no additional side effects. William eventually becomes weaker, more confused, and has difficulty swallowing. He is dying. The hospice team elects to switch William to morphine soluble tablets 15 mg every 4 hours, which Evelyn dissolves in a few drops of water and puts just inside William's lip. Indocin suppositories, 50 mg every 4 hours for anti-inflammatory effects, are added. This regimen keeps William comfortable until he dies, at which time the hospice program initiates bereavement care for Evelyn.

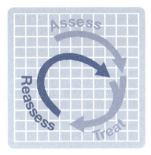

Principle Three

Reassess When Pain is Uncontrolled

- Introduction to Reassessment
- Reassess for Total Pain
- Reassess Need for Increased Involvement of Interdisciplinary Team
- Reassess Patient Compliance
- Reassess Need for Increased Dosages
  - Opioids
  - Adjuvant Drugs
- Reassess Need for Alternate Routes of Drug Administration
  - Sublingual Administration
  - Rectal Administration
  - Transdermal Administration
  - Subcutaneous Administration (SC)
  - Intravenous Administration
  - Epidural/intrathecal Administration
  - Avoid Regular Intramuscular (IM) Administration
- Reassess Need for Involvement of Other Medical Specialists

Introduction to Reassessment

Effective treatment of pain depends on careful assessment, specific interventions designed to relieve each type of pain, and continuous reassessment of the patient's pain. When pain increases or remains uncontrolled, the practitioner should institute a thorough reassessment and consider the following:

- Disease progression versus treatable complication
- Need for increased dosages of opioids and/or adjuvant drugs
- Need for alternative routes of drug administration
- Presence of unresolved emotional and spiritual pain
- Problems with patient compliance or unacceptable side effects
- Need for increased involvement of other members of interdisciplinary team and medical specialists

Reassess for Total Pain

When reassessing for total pain, it is important to focus not only on new sources of physical pain caused by disease progression or other factors, but also on nonphysical causes of pain. Reassessment may reveal painful social, emotional, or spiritual issues that were missed during the initial assessment process, or new issues may have arisen that are causing distress for the patient and/or family. The physician should initiate a gentle and thorough investigation of all possible sources of the patient's suffering.

Reassess Need for Increased Involvement of Interdisciplinary Team

During the reassessment process, the physician should consider the need for increased involvement of hospice interdisciplinary team members and other health care professionals. Important issues to explore include: Have members of the interdisciplinary team been adequately involved in caring for the patient and family? Have team members been providing effective interventions designed to relieve the suffering of this particular patient and family? Do specific members of the team need to become more involved?

Members of the Interdisciplinary Team
- Chaplain
- Team physician
- Clinical psychologist
- Enterostomal therapist
- Home health aide
- Inpatient team

- Nurse
- Physical/occupational therapist
- Pharmacist
- Registered dietitian
- Social worker/counselor
- Hospice volunteer

Reassess Patient Compliance

Because patients/family members may be embarrassed to admit noncompliance, gentle but thorough and specific questioning is needed to determine levels of compliance. Is the patient complying with recommended treatments? Are concerns about opioid treatment interfering with regular dosing at prescribed levels? Is more patient and/or family education needed? Is the patient concerned about somnolence? Constipation? Is the patient skipping doses to ensure alertness?

Reassess Need for Increased Dosages

Opioids

Is the current baseline dose still adequate to control pain? Is further titration necessary? Is a more potent opioid needed? Because no recommended dose exists that is adequa... patient, opioids *must* be in... titrated to effectively contro... appropriate titration, no ma... dose exists. Some patients may require more than 2000 mg of hydromorphone (Dilaudid) SC every day.

Adjuvant Drugs

Is an adjuvant drug needed to control pain that does not respond completely to opioid therapy? Are current doses of adjuvant drugs still adequate to control pain? Have new sources of nonopioid-responsive pain developed? Is a new class of drugs required? Should a new drug within the same class be tried? When adjuvant drugs are required, the correct dose of a strong opioid like oral morphine coupled with an effective adjuvant analgesic can provide effective relief from pain in over 90% of terminally ill patients.

Reassess Need for Alternative Routes of Drug Administration

When pain continues despite the use of effective doses of oral morphine, other routes of drug administration should be investigated because:

- The patient may not be taking the prescribed oral morphine due to difficulties with swallowing.
- The absorption of oral morphine may be inhibited, for example in the case of delayed gastric emptying.

When ambulatory patients can no longer swallow, effective alternative routes for delivering medication include the following: sublingual, rectal, transdermal, and subcutaneous (or IV if a central venous catheter is in place). Intramuscular injections are rarely necessary.

Sublingual Administration

When patients are unable to swallow, immediate-release morphine or hydromorphone (Dilaudid) can be given sublingually. The soluble morphine tablets made by Eli Lilly and concentrated oral solutions (like Roxanol) are particularly effective for sublingual administration. Lipid-soluble opioids such as fentanyl are absorbed particularly well sublingually.

Rectal Administration

When patients are unable to swallow, morphine can be given rectally. Slow-release morphine tablets (MS Contin and probably Oramorph SR) are well absorbed from the rectum and last 10-12 hours.[22] The soluble tablets made by Lilly can also be administered rectally but must be given every 4 hours in a gelatin capsule. Commercial preparations for rectal administration are available for morphine, hydromorphone, and oxymorphone. When converting from the oral to the rectal route, start with the same amount as the oral dose, then titrate as needed.

Transdermal Administration

When oral analgesics cannot be tolerated, transdermal fentanyl patches (Duragesic) can deliver 2-3 days of transdermal opioid. However, when considering the use of transdermal patches, remember the following:

- They are expensive and have a slow onset of action (12-48 hours).
- They have high variability of analgesic levels.
- They have a propensity for coming off when patients perspire.
- They require booster doses for breakthrough pain.

- They are inappropriate for patients who cannot tolerate at least 5 mg of oral morphine or its equivalent every 4 hours.
- When switching opioids, some patients will get adequate analgesia on about half the previous dose due to limited cross-tolerance.

It is important to avoid the use of patches when accurate or rapid dose titration is needed.

Use the 3:1 oral:parenteral ratio for morphine when determining potency.[23]

- Transdermal fentanyl patches (Duragesic) 25 mcg/hr = 7.5±3 mg PO morphine q 4 hours
- Transdermal fentanyl patches (Duragesic) 50 mcg/hr = 15±3 mg PO morphine q 4 hours
- Transdermal fentanyl patches (Duragesic) 75 mcg/hr = 22.5±3 mg PO morphine q 4 hours
- Transdermal fentanyl patches (Duragesic) 100 mcg/hr = 30±3 mg PO morphine q 4 hours

Because transdermal fentanyl patches (Duragesic) 100 mcg/hr provides approximately the same analgesia as 30 mg of oral morphine every 4 hours, other dose strengths can be calculated easily. For example: 1/2 of 100 mcg/hr = 50 mcg/hr and 1/2 of 30 mg = 15 mg every 4 hours.

For physicians who are accustomed to thinking in terms of 24-hour oral morphine doses, divide the 24-hour oral dose by 2 to get a rough estimate of the Duragesic equivalent, i.e., 100 mg of oral morphine/ 24 hrs is roughly equal to 50 mcg/hr Duragesic patch.

Subcutaneous Administration (SC)

Although the use of syringe drivers and other portable pumps is not yet common practice in all hospice programs in the United States, they offer a simple and effective means of pain control for many hospice patients without the pain or complications of IM or IV injections.[24] The technique is often initiated in an inpatient setting where the patient's response can be monitored carefully and the dose adjusted until optimal relief is achieved.

Patients who may benefit from continuous infusions include those with the following conditions:

- Persistent nausea and vomiting
- Severe dysphagia or swallowing disorders
- Delirium, confusion, or stupor
- High doses of oral medications that require numerous tablets

Principle Three: *Reassess When Pain is Uncontrolled*

A simple syringe driver or other portable pump can deliver subcutaneous infusions of opioids, ketorolac, and some antiemetics through a small-gauge butterfly needle into the upper chest, outer arm, thigh, abdomen, or supra-scapular region. The technique is safe, simple enough for home use, effective, inexpensive, and allows for continued patient mobility if worn in a beltlike purse or shoulder holster. Subcutaneous infusion provides blood levels comparable to those from intravenous administration. Refer to the manual that accompanies the pump for appropriate settings.

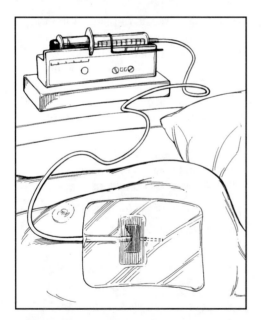

Morphine and hydromorphone are the usual drugs of choice for continuous opioid infusions. Morphine can be used in dosage strengths up to 50 mg/ml, but due to its high solubility, hydromorphone is the usual drug of choice for high dose infusions by the SC route.

- To calculate the required total daily dose of SC morphine, simply divide the patient's total daily requirement of oral morphine or equivalent by 3. For an hourly rate divide the total daily dose of SC morphine by 24 (See Tables 2 and 3).

- To calculate the required total daily dose of SC hydromorphone, simply divide the total daily oral morphine dose by 20. For an hourly rate divide the patient's total daily dose of SC hydromorphone by 24 (See Tables 2 and 3).

- Prescribe a booster dose for breakthrough pain or nausea. Usually one hour's worth of medication every 15 minutes as needed is appropriate. If more than 3-4 boosts are needed in one 8-hour period, the baseline dose should be adjusted upward.

Example:

- The patient was comfortable on 2 oxycodone with acetaminophen (Percocet) 5 mg tablets every 4 hours but now is too nauseated to tolerate PO medicines.

  – 5 mg oxycodone (one tablet) = 5 mg oral morphine

  – 10 mg oral morphine equivalent (2 tablets) X 6 doses/day = 60 mg/day

– 60 mg oral morphine/day divided by 20=3 mg SC hydromorphone/day

- Observe the patient carefully when changing opioids; due to limited cross-tolerance between opioids, some patients will require smaller doses when opioids are changed.

Note—Some patients may require as much as 500-2000 mg per day of SC hydromorphone to control their pain, so concentrated hydromorphone solutions (50-200 mg/ml) may have to be mixed from powder.

Intravenous Administration

Intravenous (IV) administration is appropriate when the patient is already receiving IV therapy for other reasons or has a central venous catheter. The intravenous route provides the most rapid onset of analgesia, but the duration of relief after a bolus dose is shorter than with other routes. Continuous intravenous infusion provides a consistent level of analgesia and is used with a small pump, as with a subcutaneous infusion. Inserting central venous catheters or restarting peripheral IVs for opioid infusion is uncomfortable and unnecessary because the subcutaneous route is equally efficacious.

Epidural/Intrathecal Administration

When the above methods do not provide acceptable relief, some carefully selected patients will benefit from a nerve block [25] or an epidural or intrathecal infusion of morphine or fentanyl, perhaps with bupivacaine or clonidine.[26]

AVOID Intramuscular (IM) Administration

This route is painful, inconvenient, and unnecessary since opioids are well absorbed subcutaneously.

Reassess Need for Involvement of Other Medical Specialists

When pain persists, consider involving the following medical specialists:
- Radiation therapist
- Neurosurgeon
- Anesthesiologist
- Medical oncologist
- Orthopedist
- Psychiatrist

These medical specialists may be able to help control pain with procedures such as:

- Limited course palliative radiation therapy
- Palliative chemotherapy
- Nerve blocks/spinal infusions
- Implantation of drug infusion systems
- Bone stabilization
- Management of severe depression or delirium
- Neurosurgical ablation

Patients need not die with unrelieved pain, even in the rare cases when the pain management methods presented in this UNIPAC are not effective. When all else fails, continuous SC or IV administration of midazolam or barbiturates can provide relaxed unconsciousness during the final days of life.[27]

Review Clinical Situation

UNIPAC Review Clinical Situation: Mildred T.

Mildred T. is a widow with multiple myeloma who lives in a nursing home. Despite several courses of melphalan (Alkeran) and prednisone, she complains of severe, all-over, deep pain. The nursing home staff reports that Mildred complains a lot, has intermittent periods of confusion, and is more depressed, irritable, and withdrawn than before. Her present medications are: hydrocodone with acetaminophen 5/500 mg (Vicodin) 1 tablet q 4 hours as needed for pain, levothyroxin 0.1 mg per day, Milk of Magnesia 30 cc as needed for constipation, docusate (Colace), and a multiple vitamin.

Review Question One

Which of the following is the appropriate course of action at this time?

[A] Order a bone scan.

[B] Prescribe morphine 10 mg PO q 4 hours.

[C] Order a serum protein electrophoresis.

[D] Prescribe an antidepressant.

[E] Take a more careful history and physical.

Correct Response and Analysis

The correct answer is E. As always, obtaining a thorough history and physical is the most appropriate action to take when first assessing a patient's multiple causes of pain.

The Case Continues: History and Physical Exam

Among other problems, the history reveals that Mildred has right hip pain on weight-bearing that eases at rest. She also has left-sided chest wall pain, particularly when she leans forward. She has been taking approximately 2 hydrocodone with acetaminophen (Vicodin) tablets per day and has had a soft bowel movement every other day. She has not taken Milk of Magnesia in more than a week. During the interview, Mildred is grumpy and withdrawn. She rates her pain as an 8 on a 10-point scale.

The physical exam reveals a very neatly dressed 68-year-old female who has just tried to arrange her snow-white hair. Mildred is of short stature with a small distance between her iliac crest and lower rib cage, suggestive of vertebral compression fractures. Her abdomen is somewhat protuberant, but she is not obese. Her extremities show some muscle wasting and trace edema in her ankles. Her legs are of equal length, and she can move all of her joints passively without discomfort. Her chest is clear, but she winces when the stethoscope is placed on the left side of her rib cage. Her skin is in good condition.

Review Question Two

The two most likely causes of Mildred's pain are:

[A] Visceral cramping

[B] Neuropathic pain

[C] Bone/soft tissue pain due to rib involvement

[D] Constipation

[E] Bone pain due to right hip involvement

Correct Response and Analysis

The correct answers are C and E. Mildred is receiving inadequate analgesic relief from the hydrocodone with acetaminophen (Vicodin), which may be due to the fact that she is not taking it on a regular around-the-clock schedule. Her aching all-over pain, coupled with rib cage tenderness, is consistent with bone/soft tissue pain due to rib involvement. The hip pain that increases on weight bearing but eases at rest is consistent with bone pain resulting from hip involvement. Mildred has had soft bowel movements every other day, and her pain does not seem to be abdominal.

The Case Continues:
Additional Information From History

Further discussion with Mildred reveals she is furious with her daughter for putting her in a nursing home and is depressed about losing her lifelong home and belongings. She particularly mourns the loss of weekly visits to her hairdresser, shopping at the mall with her friends, and the lovely clothes she used to wear. Mildred is angry with the nursing staff and now believes she is not receiving adequate care in the nursing home. Her sleep is disturbed and she refuses to swallow her medications until her pain becomes unbearable, but she will not discuss her reasons for refusing. She will not consent to an evaluation for palliative radiotherapy.

Review Question Three

At this time Mildred is experiencing physical, emotional, and social pain. Please choose the four most likely effects of her nonphysical causes of pain.

[A] They will affect medication compliance.

[B] They are likely to worsen and should be reported to the hospice social worker and counseling staff.

[C] They will exacerbate her physical pain.

[D] They will make her less likely to tolerate medication side effects.

[E] They are untreatable and will result in the need for psychiatric consultations.

Correct Response and Analysis

The correct responses are A, B, C, and D. Mildred's anger at her daughter appears to be affecting her relationship with the nursing facility staff. Both her refusal to discuss her noncompliance with medication orders and the severity of her nonphysical pain suggest the presence of complicated psychosocial issues that should be addressed by all members of the hospice team, including a social worker or other counselor. Mildred's anger and probable depression and anxiety will cause not only

Review Clinical Situation

emotional pain, they will also exacerbate her physical pain and her ability to tolerate medication side effects. They will also affect her judgment when she considers treatment options such as palliative radiation.

Review Question Four

At this time, which one of the following medications is the most appropriate choice to control Mildred's pain?

[A] Hydromorphone (Dilaudid) 2 mg PO every 4 hours

[B] Slow-release morphine 30 mg PO twice daily

[C] Transdermal fentanyl patches (Duragesic) 50 mcg /hour 1 patch q 2-3 days

[D] Hydrocodone with acetaminophen (Vicodin) 1 tablet PO every 4 hours

[E] Amitriptyline (Elavil) 50 mg PO at bedtime

Correct Response and Analysis

The correct answer is D. Hydrocodone with acetaminophen (Vicodin) 1 tablet every 4 hours is a good initial choice. Instead of switching to a more potent medication, the most appropriate action at this time is to increase the dosing frequency of the medication she is currently taking from 2 tablets a day to 1 tablet every 4 hours. The medication is not causing unacceptable side effects, she has no complaints of drowsiness, hallucinations, or itching. Constipation, a common side effect, has been addressed with a laxative.

Reminders: Hydrocodone with acetaminophen (Vicodin) 5 mg is roughly equivalent to 1-2 mg of oral morphine; an accompanying order should be written for booster doses for breakthrough pain—in this case, an appropriate order would be 1/2 tablet of hydrocodone with acetaminophen (Vicodin) every 2 hours as needed when Mildred complains of pain.

Choices A, B, C, and E are incorrect. Two milligrams of hydromorphone (Dilaudid) every 4 hours is equivalent to 8 mg of oral morphine, which is four times as potent as the hydrocodone with acetaminophen (Vicodin). In this case, such a dramatic increase in drug potency is not indicated and would probably cause unacceptable side effects.

Slow-release morphine 30 mg and transdermal fentanyl patches (Duragesic) are inappropriate for the same reasons. Although it provides smooth, continuous pain relief, slow-release morphine 30 mg every 12 hours is equivalent to 10 mg oral morphine every 4 hours, a dose that is five times as potent as the hydrocodone with acetaminophen

(Vicodin) and is likely to cause unacceptable side effects. The 50 mcg transdermal fentanyl patch (Duragesic) is equivalent to 11-18 mg of oral morphine every 4 hours, which is 5-9 times as potent as hydrocodone with acetaminophen (Vicodin). Once again, a dramatic increase in potency is not indicated and is likely to create unacceptable side effects. Amitriptyline is incorrect. Although amitriptyline can be a useful addition to an opioid analgesia regimen when treating neuropathic pain, that type of pain is not a factor in this case, and amitriptyline by itself is unlikely to provide adequate analgesia.

The Case Continues

In this case, as in most others, multiple interventions are required. The physician gently explores several issues with Mildred, including her reasons for not taking the medication on a regular basis and her anger with her daughter and the nursing home staff. Further discussion reveals that Mildred objects to taking the hydrocodone with acetaminophen (Vicodin) every 4 hours because she has known people who "got hooked" on tranquilizers and she doesn't want to become a drug addict. She thinks her daughter wants to "dope her up" so she won't complain.

The physician carefully explains the difference between physical dependence and psychological addiction, quotes medical literature about the extreme rarity of psychological addiction in cancer patients,[13] explains that the hydrocodone with acetaminophen (Vicodin) is simply counteracting the effects of the multiple myeloma, and stresses the importance of taking one hydrocodone with acetaminophen (Vicodin) on a regular 4-hour schedule. After Mildred is assured she will be able to stop taking hydrocodone with acetaminophen (Vicodin) with no problems if her pain goes away, she agrees to the 4-hour schedule.

Orders are written for 1 hydrocodone with acetaminophen (Vicodin) tablet every 4 hours on a regular basis, except at bedtime, when 2 tablets are prescribed so Mildred can skip the 2 am dose and sleep through the night. The only likely side effect of the double dose at bedtime is increased sedation, which is desirable at night.

After switching to the new regime, Mildred discovers that her pain is adequately controlled at rest, but she continues to experience severe pain in her hip when she tries to get out of bed and walk. Additional booster doses before getting out of bed do not control the pain on walking. The nurse and social worker report that Mildred's depressive symptoms have begun to improve following the relief of pain and talks with the hospice counselor.

Review Clinical Situation

Adequate pain control and counseling help alleviate interpersonal problems that appeared deeply rooted and resistant to intervention. With the help of the hospice counselor, Mildred is able to reflect on several issues, including her long-term relationship with her daughter, her daughter's fight for independence, and her own feelings of rejection. As Mildred's psychosocial and physical pain are controlled, her suffering decreases.

Review Question Five

Which one of the following is the best choice for controlling Mildred's pain on movement?

[A] Transdermal fentanyl patches (Duragesic) 50 mcg per hour 1 patch q 3 days

[B] Physical therapy for progressive ambulation exercises

[C] Oxycodone and acetaminophen (Percocet) 1-2 tablets every 4 hours plus ibuprofen 400 mg every 4 hours

[D] Amitriptyline at bedtime in addition to the hydrocodone with acetaminophen (Vicodin)

[E] Slow-release morphine 30 mg every 8 hours

Correct Response and Analysis

The correct answer is C. Pain that occurs only on movement can be difficult to control because the amount of analgesic necessary to control pain on movement may be too much at rest. Because Mildred is comfortable at rest, a dramatic increase in dose is likely to cause increased side effects. Oxycodone and acetaminophen (Percocet) offers a moderate increase in potency and ibuprofen is an appropriate adjuvant drug for bone/soft tissue pain that may add additional analgesia without compromising her mental status.

If pain persists despite the use of ibuprofen, a brief course of palliative radiation therapy may relieve Mildred's pain if she has not already received radiation to that area and agrees to the treatment. Transdermal fentanyl patches (Duragesic) and slow-release morphine are incorrect. Even though the increased opioid dose might be helpful when she is up and moving, the same dose is likely to cause excessive drowsiness and confusion while at rest. Amitriptyline is incorrect. As an adjuvant, amitriptyline is much more likely to help relieve neuropathic pain than bone/soft tissue pain. In this case, neuropathic pain is not an issue, and Mildred's depressive symptoms are already resolving.

The Case Continues

When the physician visits the nursing home again, Mildred is using her walker to walk down the hall. She is grateful for the physician's efforts to control her pain but says she doesn't have time to talk because a bridge game is starting in a few minutes. Mildred mentions mild discomfort on movement but says it is not enough to keep her immobile. She doesn't want to bother with radiation therapy.

Mildred enjoys 6 weeks of good pain control during which time her strength gradually declines. Her ibuprofen is decreased due to stomach upset, but otherwise her symptoms remain under good control.

One day Mildred develops a temperature, becomes too weak to get out of bed, has difficulty swallowing her ibuprofen and oxycodone and acetaminophen (Percocet) tablets, and is unable to respond with more than one syllable when the nurse asks her a question. The physician examines her and suspects pneumonia or a urinary tract infection, and discusses the situation with Mildred and her daughter. A decision is made to withhold antibiotic treatment because Mildred's condition appears to be part of the natural course of her myeloma and she has always insisted she does not want the debilitating stage of her disease to be prolonged.

Mildred has been taking 2 oxycodone and acetaminophen (Percocet) tablets every 4 hours and 400 mg ibuprofen every 8 hours but is now unable to swallow such large pills.

Review Clinical Situation

Review Question Six

Which of the following will provide pain relief in a simple but effective manner?

[A] Slow release morphine 30 tablet mg every 12 hours PO or per rectum

[B] Transdermal fentanyl patch (Duragesic) 50 mcg per hour 1 patch every 3 days with Indocin 50 mg q 12 hours per rectum

[C] IV morphine at 5 mg per hour

[D] PCA pump delivering hydromorphone (Dilaudid) at 0.5 mg per hour (basal rate) with 0.5 mg q 30 minutes prn (PCA)

[E] Transfer to hospital for further evaluation

Correct Response and Analysis

The best responses are either A or B. The transdermal fentanyl patch (Duragesic) provides an oral morphine equivalent of 11-18 mg every 4 hours, which is less than a 50% increase over the oxycodone and acetaminophen (Percocet), is non-invasive, does not require the ability to swallow tablets, and is much easier to manage than an IV or PCA pump in a nursing home situation. Slow-release morphine (MS Contin and probably Oramorph SR) tablets are absorbed rectally about as well as by mouth. In either case, sublingual morphine 5 mg as needed would be an adequate booster dose.

Incorrect responses are C, D, and E. A continuous IV infusion of morphine at 5 mg per hour is the equivalent of 60 mg of oral morphine every 4 hours, a dose that is much too potent and is likely to cause confusion and could result in Mildred's attempting to pull out the peripheral line. This route is also difficult to manage in a nursing home.

A PCA pump also requires a peripheral IV unless it is delivered subcutaneously, but requiring Mildred to punch a button to control pain is neither realistic nor appropriate given her fever and decreasing mental status.

A transfer is unnecessary because Mildred's symptoms can be adequately controlled in the nursing home. In addition, a decision has been made to forgo aggressive treatment of the complications of her myeloma so there is no need for acute care. Mildred does not want the debilitating stage of her illness to be prolonged, and she might get less pain relief in a hospital.

The Case Concludes

Using these measures, Mildred is able to remain in the nursing home in relative comfort. She develops rattling secretions that are controlled with 2 scopolamine patches (Transderm Scop) and dies comfortably 2 days later in the presence of her daughter. Mildred's daughter and the nursing home staff are grateful for the hospice/palliative care interventions.

NOTE—Although the tendency among many physicians is to classify every psychosocial problem as a mental health issue and immediately write a prescription for a psychoactive drug or make a psychiatric referral, other actions may be more appropriate. Before prescribing medication to relieve mild to moderate anxiety and depression, the practitioner should first attempt nondrug measures, such as facilitating good communication that includes careful listening and brief counseling. During the communication process, physicians should be sensitive to the severity of the patient's psychosocial or spiritual problems and to their own levels of competence, and, when necessary, refer the patient to other members of the interdisciplinary team or to an outside specialist.

Physicians and patients vary in their willingness to talk about psychosocial and spiritual issues. When patients and their physicians want to discuss such issues, the physician should schedule enough time to sit down and thoroughly explore troubling issues. When physicians are uncomfortable talking about spiritual or psychological issues, patients should be referred to other members of the interdisciplinary team, such as the social worker, counselor, chaplain, or volunteer. However, in this case, the physician's initial assessment may be a valuable addition to assessments made by other team members. By working together, health care professionals are more likely to offer effective interventions that relieve not just physical pain but also the pain caused by spiritual and psychosocial issues.

Test Clinical Situation

Please see correct responses on the answer sheet that follows.

Test Clinical Situation: Dennis and Jean D.

Dennis D. is a male dentist with carcinoma of the stomach who has just been referred for hospice/palliative care. He has had several courses of chemotherapy, none of which slowed the progression of his disease. He is taking the following medications: 30 mg of slow-release morphine twice a day, 25 mg of chlorpromazine (Thorazine) three times a day for nausea, 50 mg of amitriptyline (Elavil) at bedtime for sleep, and 2 senna 5 mg plus docusate 100 mg (Senokot S) tablets twice daily for constipation.

During the physician's assessment visit to Dennis and Jean's beautifully appointed home, Dennis complains of abdominal pain that he describes as 7.2 overall on a 10-point scale. He says the pain sometimes feels cramping and fluctuates from a 3 to a 9 depending on whether or not he has just urinated.

TEST Question One

At this point, which one of the following is the most appropriate course of action?

[A] Increase the dose of slow-release morphine.

[B] Order a CT scan of the abdomen.

[C] Order a gastrostomy.

[D] Order a complete blood count.

[E] Complete a history and physical examination.

History and Physical Exam

The history reveals a man who feels the need to urinate almost hourly throughout the day and night and requires his wife's assistance to walk from their bed to the bathroom. Both Dennis and Jean are exhausted from interrupted sleep and the physical difficulty of making such frequent trips to the bathroom. Dennis has had a moderate-size bowel movement each day during the past 7 days.

Test Clinical Situation

The physical exam reveals a bald, 42-year-old male with a clear chest, an abdomen that is tender in the upper quadrants with a rock-hard mass in the epigastric area, and a large round mass just above the pubis. His extremities show muscle wasting and trace edema.

TEST Question Two

Three likely causes of Dennis's lower abdominal pain are:

[A] Tumor involvement of viscera

[B] Ureteral obstruction by tumor

[C] Urinary retention

[D] Poor medication compliance

[E] Medication side effects

Note—Consider the combined anticholinergic effects of morphine, chlorpromazine (Thorazine), and amitriptyline (Elavil).

The Case Continues: Additional Information From History

Further discussion reveals that Dennis is anguished about leaving his two young children without a father and is very concerned about his rapidly decreasing ability to function physically. When Jean leaves the room, the physician asks if anything else is troubling him and Dennis begins to weep quietly. He reveals a troubled marriage that was further threatened by an affair he had just before he became ill. Dennis has been active in his church and questions whether his illness is a punishment for his affair. He is overwhelmed with guilt and hates having to constantly rely on his wife.

TEST Question Three

Which three of the following types of nonphysical pain appear to be causing distress in this case?

[A] Emotional pain

[B] Neuropathic pain

[C] Social pain

[D] Spiritual pain

[E] Financial pain

TEST Question Four

Which three responses best describe how nonphysical pain is likely to affect the course of Dennis' illness?

[A] It is irrelevant to the treatment and management of this case.

[B] It is likely to effect Dennis' acceptance of the catheter he may need to relieve his urinary retention.

[C] It is unlikely he will be able to tolerate the withdrawal of the chlorpromazine and amitriptyline that are causing his urinary retention unless other medications are prescribed to treat his anxiety and depression.

[D] It is likely to greatly exaggerate his suffering regardless of medication.

[E] A psychiatric referral will be necessary.

The Case Continues

The chlorpromazine (Thorazine) and amitriptyline (Elavil) are discontinued, and haloperidol (Haldol) 1 mg twice daily is substituted for control of nausea, with lorazepam 1 mg at bedtime to help with sleep. Dennis' urinary retention subsides, but he still complains of moderate amounts of upper abdominal pain. The physician and nurse agree that this pain seems to be the result of tumor involvement of his stomach, so the physician increases the slow-release morphine to 30 mg three times a day. Note: Slow release morphine tablets usually last 12 hours but may be prescribed every 8 hours to evenly distribute 90 mg of morphine over 24 hours.

The increased dose of slow-release morphine helps temporarily but causes unacceptable amounts of drowsiness. Without consulting the physician, Dennis reduces his slow-release morphine dose to 30 mg twice daily with the return of unacceptable levels of pain.

TEST Question Five

Which one of the following is the best course of action to relieve Dennis's pain?

[A] Continue the slow-release morphine with instructions that Dennis must take it if he wants good pain relief.

[B] Give 15 mg of immediate release morphine every 4 hours with 10 mg morphine every 2 hours if needed for breakthrough pain.

[C] Add doxepin (Sinequan) 50 mg at bedtime.

[D] Switch from morphine to hydromorphone (Dilaudid) 4 mg every 4 hours with 2 mg hydromorphone every 2 hours if needed.

[E] Start a morphine drip at 2 mg per hour, with 1 mg every 30 minutes if needed.

The Case Continues

The physician asks Dennis to try the new medication but warns him that a change in medication might cause drowsiness for a day or two. Dennis reluctantly agrees, and 3 days later his wife reports that Dennis is mentally clear, much more comfortable, and able to urinate. With the help of the hospice chaplain, Dennis and Jean make progress with giving and receiving forgiveness, which further increases his comfort. However, as the weeks pass, Dennis' strength continues to deteriorate, and he becomes bedbound and intermittently confused. The pain in his abdomen begins to require frequent booster doses of the new medication, and one night his wife has to give him additional doses every 2 hours throughout the night. He is having great difficulty swallowing tablets.

TEST Question Six

At this time, which one of the following is the most appropriate (effective and least invasive) course of action?

[A] Transfer Dennis to the hospital for a celiac plexus block.

[B] Insert an epidural catheter for epidural morphine infusion.

[C] Begin an SC infusion of hydromorphone (Dilaudid) at 8 mg per day.

[D] Begin a PCA pump with hydromorphone (Dilaudid) at 1 mg every 15 minutes as needed.

[E] Tell Jean that Dennis' confusion is expected and she should carry on as before.

The Case Continues

Jean calls the next day to report that Dennis' pain is well controlled and that both of them were able to sleep. Several days later, she calls again to report that Dennis has become restless and agitated and is calling out to people who are not there. Jean is very distressed by this new symptom. All efforts to talk with Dennis about what is going on are unsuccessful because he is unable to concentrate on the questions.

TEST Question Seven

Which of the following interventions would be appropriate at this time?

[A] Double the infusion dose of hydromorphone (Dilaudid).

[B] Add haloperidol (Haldol) 5 mg per day and midazolam (Versed) 5 mg per day to the hydromorphone (Dilaudid) infusion, *or* use chlorpromazine (Thorazine) 50-100 mg suppositories per rectum q 4-6 hours as needed.

[C] Transfer Dennis to a hospice inpatient unit for aggressive palliative care.

[D] Discontinue the opioid analgesic.

[E] Order secobarbital (Seconal) tablets #50 and let Jean know that Dennis will die if she gives all of them to him.

The Case Concludes

Dennis dies 2 days later from natural causes, and Jean is grateful for the hospice/palliative care interventions. For more information on physician-assisted suicide and euthanasia, see *UNIPAC Six: Ethical and Legal Decision Making When Caring for the Terminally Ill.*

Test Clinical Situation Correct Responses

1) E is correct because completing a thorough history and physical is the most appropriate action to take when first assessing a patient's multiple causes of pain. The other responses are incorrect because the physician does not yet have enough information to make decisions about changes in treatment.

2) A, C, and E are correct because Dennis has a rock-hard mass consistent with tumor involvement of the viscera that is likely to be causing pain, and the combined anticholinergic side effects of morphine, chlorpromazine (Thorazine), and amitriptyline (Elavil) are likely to be causing urinary retention. B and D are incorrect because Dennis' bladder contains urine and he is complying with the medication orders.

3) A, C, and D are the most appropriate responses because Dennis has voiced feelings of guilt, anguish about leaving two small children, and concerns about being punished for his behavior. B is incorrect because neuropathic pain is not a nonphysical cause of pain and because Dennis does not describe his pain as "burning," "shooting," or "stabbing." E is less likely to be correct than the other responses because Dennis has not yet voiced any financial concerns and he appears to have adequate financial resources.

4) B is correct because a catheter may be viewed by Dennis as one more sign of his increasing dependence or as a symbol of punishment for his affair. C and D are correct because Dennis is likely to need medication to treat anxiety and depression and because nonphysical pain contributes to total pain and exacerbates suffering. Response A is incorrect because the components of total pain are interactive—Dennis' emotional, spiritual, and social pain are likely to exacerbate his physical pain. E is incorrect because Dennis' nonphysical causes of pain can likely be alleviated with effective symptom control and support from the hospice team.

5) D is correct because rotating opioids may reduce unacceptable side effects. Response A is incorrect because attempts should be made to alleviate distressing side effects. B, C, and E are incorrect because they are unlikely to reduce drowsiness. The opioid doses are higher than was acceptable to Dennis, and doxepin can be quite sedating when first used.

6) C is correct because Dennis' increased pain indicates disease progression and the need for opioid dosages high enough to effectively control pain. Responses A and B are incorrect because Dennis' pain can likely be controlled without resorting to such invasive measures, D is incorrect because Dennis' weakness and confusion will interfere with his ability to operate a PCA pump, and E is incorrect because attempts should be made to alleviate the distressing symptom of confusion.

7) B or C are correct because either haloperidol and midazolam OR chlorpromazine are likely to relieve Dennis' agitation, and admission to a hospice inpatient unit may be the most appropriate setting for controlling severe agitation and relieving family stress. A is incorrect because increasing the infusion dose of hydromorphone is unlikely to reduce Dennis' agitation, D is incorrect because it is likely to result in high levels of pain, and E is incorrect because other less drastic and final solutions are likely to control Dennis' symptoms, and are less likely to contribute to possible complicated grief reactions for the bereaved.

Pretest Correct Responses

1. **True.** In addition, the pain usually follows the distribution of a sensory nerve. (See page 12)

2. **True.** The World Health Organization's 3-step ladder has been proven to be an effective way to control pain in a high percentage of cancer patients. (See page 25)

3. **False.** Meperidine has a low oral potency and a toxic metabolite that can cause tremors and seizures. (See page 33)

4. **False.** Neuropathic pain may respond partially to opioids, but adjuvant drugs like antidepressants or anticonvulsants are usually necessary. (See page 38)

5. **False.** Pain and dyspnea seem to antagonize the sedative and respiratory depressant effects of opioids. (See page 21)

6. **True.** This simple, noninvasive route is an effective way to deliver opioids. (See page 55)

7. **True.** Most of the important information needed to effectively relieve pain can be obtained from a history and physical examination. (See page 8)

8. **True.** When morphine is prescribed in effective doses, its analgesic effects last about 4 hours. If the patient is only receiving 2-3 hours of pain relief, increase the dose to extend the duration of action. (See page 31)

9. **False.** Supportive counseling and a multi-disciplinary approach to symptom control can provide excellent relief for some patients with mild to moderate depression; however, pharmacologic therapy must be considered when anxiety and depression are severe and do not respond to these efforts. (See page 43)

10. **True.** Constipation is a very common side effect of opioid therapy and should be anticipated. (See page 33)

11. **False.** When patients are in severe pain, the daily dose of morphine may have to be titrated upward rapidly. (See page 31)

12. **True.** Low to full doses of a tricyclic antidepressant like amitriptyline can help relieve neuropathic pain. (See page 38)

13. **True.** Learning to calculate equivalent doses of different opioids is an important skill in hospice/palliative care. (See Table 3 on page 28)

14. **True.** For example, morphine is not the drug of choice for treating constipation. (See page 24)

15. **True.** Oxycodone is comparable in potency to oral morphine. (See Table 2 on page 26)

16. **True.** In addition to the patient's regularly scheduled maintenance dose, "booster" or "rescue" doses are provided on an as-needed basis to help relieve increases in pain that can accompany short periods of stress or activity. (See page 32)

17. **True.** Listening to the adjectives patients use to describe their pain can help differentiate cancer-related pains so type-specific treatments can be initiated. Bone pain may require the addition of a NSAID or another adjuvant drug for complete relief. (See page 12)

18. **True.** Effective treatment of this distressing pain is greatly appreciated and often requires both an opioid and an anticholinergic. (See page 39)

19. **True.** This is a useful alternative route for delivering opioids to patients who can not swallow tablets. (See page 27)

20. **True.** These are the components of "Total Pain," a term used to describe the all-encompassing pain often experienced by terminally ill patients. (See page 12)

Posttest

AAHPM

Please read each item and circle the one correct response to each item on the detachable answer sheet at the back of the book.

Please read each item and circle the one correct response to each item on the detachable answer sheet at the back of the book.

1. (Complete the blank) Studies indicate that more than _____ % of the cancer pain experienced by terminally ill patients can be effectively controlled using currently available therapies. (See page 6)

[A] 20

[B] 90

[C] 50

[D] 15

2. Patients usually describe neuropathic pain as: (See page 12)

[A] Shooting or burning

[B] Cramping

[C] Deep and aching

[D] Dull

3. Patients often describe bone pain as: (See page 12)

[A] Shooting

[B] Deep and aching

[C] Spasms or cramping

[D] Colicky

4. Which of the following classes of drugs can be effective adjuvants to morphine when treating specific types of pain? (See page 38-39)

[A] NSAIDs

[B] Antidepressants

[C] Anticholinergics

[D] All of the above

5. To calculate an effective initial daily dose of subcutaneous hydromorphone (Dilaudid), divide the patient's daily dose of oral morphine by: (See page 28)

[A] 20

[B] 3

[C] 5

[D] 2

6. When titrating morphine, the dose can never be raised by more than 25% over a 24-hour period. (See page 31)

[A] True

[B] False

7. When bone pain occurs, which of the following may be an effective adjuvant to morphine? (See page 38)

   [A] Ibuprofen

   [B] Naproxen

   [C] Indomethacin

   [D] All of the above

8. To calculate the equivalent daily parenteral dose of 30 mg of oral morphine, divide the oral dose of morphine by 3. (See page 28)

   [A] True

   [B] False

9. When titrating morphine, the most appropriate booster or increment dose for a patient receiving a baseline dose of 30 mg every 4 hours is: (See page 32)

   [A] 2-5 mg

   [B] 10-15 mg

   [C] 20-39 mg

   [D] None of the above

10. When pain related to nerve damage or dysesthesia occurs, which of the following may be an effective adjuvant to morphine: (See page 38)

    [A] Amitriptyline (Elavil)

    [B] Scopolamine

    [C] Doxepin (Sinequan)

    [D] A and C above

11. A patient is receiving 60 mg of oral morphine per day. The equivalent daily dose of parenteral hydromorphone (Dilaudid) is: (See page 28)

    [A] 30 mg

    [B] 20 mg

    [C] 5 mg

    [D] 3 mg

12. Due to concerns about addiction, tolerance, and decreased respiration, the use of morphine or other strong opioids should be saved for the last few weeks or days of the patient's life. (See page 22)

    [A] True

    [B] False

13. Completing a history and physical are the first steps of an effective assessment of all types of pain. (See page 8)

   [A] True

   [B] False

14. When the common side effect of constipation occurs as a result of opioid therapy, an appropriate first step is to find out what laxative the patient has been using and how effective it has been. (See page 34)

   [A] True

   [B] False

15. Most terminally ill patients on opioid therapy require individually titrated doses of potent bowel stimulants such as: (See page 34)

   [A] Senna (Senokot)

   [B] Bisacodyl (Dulcolax)

   [C] Either A or B above

   [D] Docusate (Colace)

16. Four types of pain can contribute to a patient's experience of total pain: physical, emotional, social, and spiritual pain. (See page 12)

   [A] True

   [B] False

17. When a patient can no longer swallow, which of the following are appropriate alternative routes of opioid administration for ambulatory patients: (See page 54)

   [A] Sublingual

   [B] Subcutaneous

   [C] Intramuscular

   [D] Both A and B above

18. Corticosteroids, such as dexamethasone, are effective adjuvants to morphine when treating pain caused by raised intracranial pressure. (See page 39)

   [A] True

   [B] False

19. The correct dose of a strong opioid like oral morphine and an adjuvant analgesic provide effective relief from pain in more than 90% of terminally ill patients. (See page 25)

   [A] True

   [B] False

20. Meperidine (Demerol) is often the analgesic of choice in the hospice/palliative care setting. (See page 33)

   [A] True

   [B] False

21. Morphine usually relieves neuropathic pain without the use of adjuvant drugs. (See page 12)

   [A] True

   [B] False

22. Clinically significant respiratory depression is a common result of opioid use. (See page 21)

   [A] True

   [B] False

23. An effective dose of immediate-release oral morphine provides about 4 hours of pain relief. (See page 31)

   [A] True

   [B] False

24. All terminally ill patients with severe depression should receive psychological and/or pharmacological treatment. (See page 43)

   [A] True

   [B] False

25. Nearly all patients receiving opioid therapy should be placed on a laxative regimen to prevent constipation. (See page 33)

   [A] True

   [B] False

26. One 100 mcg/hr transdermal fentanyl patch (Duragesic) equals approximately 30±3 mg PO morphine q 4 hours. (See page 55)

   [A] True

   [B] False

27. Effective pain management is dependent on an effective assessment of the causes of noncancer-related pain, cancer-related pain, and nonphysical pain. (See page 8)

   [A] True

   [B] False

28. One oxycodone and acetaminophen (Percocet) tablet is roughly the equivalent of 5 mg of oral morphine. (See page 26)

   [A] True

   [B] False

29. Visceral spasm pain can be effectively treated with an opioid and an anticholinergic, such as scopolamine. (See page 39)

   [A] True

   [B] False

30. Soluble tablets can provide effective sublingual delivery of morphine. (See page 27)

   [A] True

   [B] False

References

[1] Jacox A, Carr DB, Payne R, et al. *Management of Cancer Pain. Clinical Practice Guideline No. 9.* AHCPR Publication N. 94-0592. Rockville, MD. Agency for Health Care Policy and Research, U.S. Department of Health and Human Services, Public Health Service; March 1994:8.

[2] Twycross R. Evaluation. In: Twycross R. *Pain Relief in Advanced Cancer.* New York: Churchill Livingston; 1994:111-128.

[3] Anand A, Carmosino L. Glatt, AE. Evaluation of recalcitrant pain in HIV-infected hospitalized patients. *J Acquired Imm D Synd.* 1994;7:52-56.

[4] Foley KM. Pain assessment and cancer pain syndromes. In: Doyle D, Hanks GW, MacDonald N, eds. *Oxford Textbook of Palliative Medicine.* New York: Oxford University Press; 1993:148-165.

[5] Beyer JE, Wells N. Assessment of cancer pain in children. In: Patt RB, ed. *Cancer Pain.* Philadelphia: JB Lippincott; 1993:57-84.

[6] Breitbart W, Patt RB. Pain management in the patient with AIDS. *Heme/Onc Annals.* 1994;2(6):391-399.

[7] Foley KM. Management of cancer pain. In: DeVita VT, Hellman S, Rosenberg SA, eds. *Cancer: Principles and Practice of Oncology.* 4th ed. Philadelphia: Lippincott; 1993:2417-2448.

[8] Twycross R. Misunderstandings about morphine. In: Twycross R. *Pain Relief in Advanced Cancer.* New York: Churchill Livingston; 1994:333-347.

[9] Bruera E, MacMillan K, Pither J, MacDonald RN. Effects of morphine on the dyspnea of terminal cancer patients. *J Pain Symptom Manage.* 1990;5:341-344.

[10] Bruera E, MacEachern T, Ripamonti C, Hanson J. Subcutaneous morphine for dyspnea in cancer patients. *Ann Intern Med.* 1993;119:906-907.

[11] Light RW, Muro JR, Sato RI, Stansbury DW, Fischer CE, Brown SE. Effects of oral morphine on breathlessness and exercise tolerance in patients with chronic obstructive pulmonary disease. *Am Rev Respir Dis.* 1989;139:126-133.

[12] Porter J, Jick H., Boston Collaborative Drug Surveillance Program. Addiction rare in patients treated with narcotics. *N Engl J Med.* 1980;302(2):123.

[13] Hanks GWC, Portenoy RK, MacDonald N, O'Neill WM. Difficult pain problems. In: Doyle D, Hanks GW, MacDonald N, eds. *Oxford Textbook of Palliative Medicine.* New York: Oxford University Press; 1993:257-274.

[14] Robb V. Working on the edge: palliative care for substance users with AIDS. *J Palliat Care.* 1995;11(2);50-53.

[15] Gonzales GR, Coyle N. Treatment of cancer pain in a former opioid abuser: fears of the patient and staff and their influence on care. *J Pain Symptom Manage.* 1992;7(4):246-249.

[16] Lederle FA, Busch DL, Mattox KM, West MJ, Aske DM. Cost-effective treatment of constipation in the elderly: a randomized double-blind comparison of sorbitol and lactulose. *Am J Med.* 1990;89:597-601.

[17] DeConno F, Zecca E, Martini C, Ripamonti C, Caraceni A, Saita L. Tolerability of ketorolac administered via continuous subcutaneous infusion for cancer pain: a preliminary report. *J Pain Symptom Manage.* 1994;9(2):119-121.

[18] Portenoy RK. Adjuvant analgesics in pain management. In: Doyle D, Hanks GW, MacDonald N, eds. *Oxford Textbook of Palliative Medicine.* New York: Oxford University Press: 1993:187-203.

[19] Storey P, Trumble M. Rectal doxepin and carbamazepine therapy in patients with cancer. *N Engl J Med.* 1992;327:1318-1319.

[20] Cassel EJ. The nature of suffering and the goals of medicine. *N Engl J Med.* 1982;306(11):639-645.

[21] Billings JA. Palliative medicine update: depression. *J Palliat Care.* 1995;11(1):48-54.

[22] Wilkinson TJ, Robinson BA, Begg EJ, Duffull SB, Ravenscroft PJ, Schneider JJ. Pharmacokinetics and efficacy of rectal versus oral sustained release morphine in cancer patients. *Cancer Chemother Pharmacol.* 1992;31:251-254.

[23] Storey P. More on the conversion of transdermal fentanyl to morphine. *J Pain Symptom Manage.* 1995;10(8):581.

[24] Storey P, Hill HH, St. Louis RH, Tarver EE. Subcutaneous infusions for control of cancer symptoms. *J Pain Symptom Manage.* 1990;5:33-41.

[25] Raj PP. Local anesthetic blockade. In: Patt RB, ed. *Cancer Pain.* Philadelphia: Lippincott; 1993:329-341.

[26] Devulder J, Ghys L. Dhondt W, Rolly G. Spinal analgesia in terminal care: risk versus benefit. *J Pain Symptom Manage.* 1994;9(2):75-81.

[27] Cherny NI, Portenoy RK. Sedation in the management of refractory symptoms: guidelines for evaluation and treatment. *J Palliat Care.* 1994;10(2):31-38.

Notes

Posttest: Answer Sheet

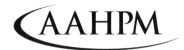

UNIPAC Three: Assessment and Treatment of Pain in the Terminally Ill

Physicians are eligible to receive 3 credit hours in Category 1 of the AMA/PRA by completing and returning this posttest answer sheet to the AAHPM. The Academy will keep a record of AMA/PRA Category 1 credit hours and the record will be provided on request; however, physicians are responsible for reporting their own Category 1 CME credits when applying for the AMA/PRA or for other certificates or credentials.

Name

Street

City/State/Zip Code

Telephone

Social Security Number

Please mail this answer sheet and a check payable to *"AAHPM"* in the amount of:

$45.00 — *AAHPM members*
$60.00 — *non-members*

Physician Training Programs
American Academy of Hospice
 and Palliative Medicine
PO Box 14288
Gainesville, FL 32604-2288

Please circle the one correct answer for each question. For true/false items, circle A if the correct response is "true" and circle B if the correct response is "false."

1. A	B	C	D		16. A	B		
2. A	B	C	D		17. A	B	C	D
3. A	B	C	D		18. A	B		
4. A	B	C	D		19. A	B		
5. A	B	C	D		20. A	B		
6. A	B				21. A	B		
7. A	B	C	D		22. A	B		
8. A	B				23. A	B		
9. A	B	C	D		24. A	B		
10. A	B	C	D		25. A	B		
11. A	B	C	D		26. A	B		
12. A	B				27. A	B		
13. A	B				28. A	B		
14. A	B				29. A	B		
15. A	B	C	D		30. A	B		

Notes

Notes

Notes

Table 2

Oral Morphine Equivalents

Oral Morphine Equivalent	Easiest to Swallow	Also Useful	Notes
1-2 mg	codeine soluble tablet* 30 mg	APAP** + Codeine 30 mg (Tylenol #3)	• Codeine with APAP and hydrocodone are the **only** drugs on this list that **do not require a triplicate prescription** (in states that require them).
	oxycodone elixir 1cc (5 mg/5 cc)	hydrocodone 5 mg (Hycodan)	
5 mg	oxycodone elixir 5 cc (5 mg/5 cc)	oxycodone 5 mg + APAP 325 mg (Percocet)	• Oxycodone is rarely nauseating.
	morphine dissolve 10 mg soluble tablet in 2 cc of water and give 1cc	oxycodone 5 mg + APAP 500 mg (Tylox)	• Avoid hepatic APAP toxicity by limiting APAP dose to <1000 mg (3 Percocet or 2 Tylox) every 4 hrs.
10 mg	morphine 10 mg soluble tablet	morphine 10 mg/ 5cc syrup	• Syrup is too dilute for use at higher doses.
	hydromorphone (Dilaudid) 2.5 mg tablets	morphine 30 mg slow-release tabs, 1 q 12 hrs. (MS Contin 30 mg or Oramorph SR 30 mg)	• Slow-release tablets are not useful for booster doses.
15 mg (= 5 mg IM morphine)	morphine 15 mg soluble tablet	morphine 30 mg slow-release tabs, 1 q 8 hrs. (MS Contin 30 mg or Oramorph SR 30 mg)	• Do not crush slow-release tablets.
20 mg	hydromorphone (Dilaudid) 5 mg	morphine 20 mg/cc solution 1 ml (Roxanol)	• Concentrated liquids require careful measuring.
30 mg (=10 mg IM morphine)	morphine 30 mg soluble tablet	Higher doses from multiples of the above. (Oramorph MS Contin) 60 mg 1 tab every 8 hrs	* Soluble tablets are immediate-release with rapid dissolution times. ** APAP = acetaminophen

Copyright © 1996 American Academy of Hospice and Palliative Medicine, extracted from *UNIPAC Three: Assessment and Treatment of Pain in the Terminally Ill* by P. Storey & C. Knight. The American Academy of Hospice and Palliative Medicine, P.O. Box 14288, Gainesville, FL 32604 (352) 377-8900

Table 9

Suggested Adjuvant Drug Dosages

Pain Source	Pain Character	Drug Class	Examples	Notes
Bone or soft tissue	Tenderness over bone or joint, especially on movement	NSAIDs	Ibuprofen 400 mg PO q 4 hr	Inexpensive, big pills
			Sulindac (Clinoril) 200 PO mg q 12 hrs	Well tolerated, preferred in renal impairmen
			Naproxen (Naprosyn Susp) 125 mg/5cc, 15 cc PO q 8-12 hrs	Liquid preparation available
			Indomethacin (Indocin 50 mg) caps or supp. q 8 hrs	Suppository, may cause more gastritis
			Piroxicam (Feldene 20 mg) capsules, 1 PO qd	Easiest to swallow, may cause more gastritis
			Choline Mg trisalicylate (Trilisate susp) 500 mg/5cc, 15 cc q 12	Preferred in thrombocytopenia
Nerve damage or dysesthesia	Burning or scalding pain	Tricyclic antidepressants	Amitriptyline (Elavil) 10-100 PO mg q hs	Best studied, sedating, start with low dose
			Doxepin (Sinequan) 10-100 mg PO q hs	10 mg/cc susp. available
			Trazodone (Desyrel) 25-150 mg PO q hs	+Less anticholinergic effect, 1/3 as potent as amitriptyline
	Shooting, stabbing pain	Anticonvulsants	Carbamazepine (Tegretol) 200 mg PO q 6-12 hrs Valproate (Depakote) 250 mg PO tid-qid	Both are absorbed from rectum
Visceral spasms	Colic, cramping abdominal pain, bladder spasms	Anticholinergics	Scopolamine (Transderm Scop) 1-2 patches q 3d	Scopolamine may also be mixed with narcotic in SC infusion 0.8-2.4 mg/d
			Hyoscyamine (Levsin) 0.125 mg PO or SL q 4-8 hrs	Capsules, SL tabs, or liquid
			Oxybutynin (Ditropan) 5-10 mg PO q 8 hrs	Tablets or liquid

Copyright © 1996 American Academy of Hospice and Palliative Medicine, extracted from *UNIPAC Three: Assessment and Treatment of Pain in the Terminally Ill* by P. Storey & C. Knight. The American Academy of Hospice and Palliative Medicine, P.O. Box 14288, Gainesville, FL 32604 (352) 377-8900